MIRIAM E. NELSON, PH.D.

with Sarah Wernick, Ph.D.

STRONG WOMEN

STAY YOUNG

REVISED EDITION

Illustrations by Wendy Wray

BANTAM BOOKS

NEW YORK TORONTO

LONDON SYDNEY AUCKLAND

STRONG WOMEN STAY YOUNG

PUBLISHING HISTORY
Bantam hardcover edition / February 1997
Bantam trade paperback edition / January 1998
Bantam revised trade paperback edition / April 2000

Graph on page 31 reprinted with permission from Morganti et al.,
Med Sci Sports Exerc 1995; 27 (6) 906–12.
Photos on page 48 reprinted with permission from Dempster et al.,
J Bone Min Res 1986; 1:15–21.

The research described in this book has been funded at least in part with federal funds from the U.S.
Department of Agriculture, Agricultural Research Service. The contents of this publication do not
necessarily reflect the views or policies of the U.S. Department of Agriculture, nor does mention of
trade names, commercial products, or organizations imply endorsement by the U.S. Government.

Library of Congress Catalog Card Number 96-41541

ISBN 0-553-38077-X

Published simultaneously in the United States and Canada

Bantam Books are published by Bantam Books, a division of Random House, Inc. Its trademark,
consisting of the words "Bantam Books" and the portrayal of a rooster, is Registered in U.S. Patent and
Trademark Office and in other countries. Marca Registrada. Bantam Books, 1540 Broadway, New York,
New York 10036.

PRINTED IN THE UNITED STATES OF AMERICA

BVG 10   9   8   7   6   5   4   3   2   1

Readers rave about *Strong Women Stay Young*

"I consider myself very fit and healthy. I cycle an eleven-mile route (with hills) three to four times a week and walk two to two and a half miles the remaining days. Your strength-training program sounded like a manageable addition to my fitness routine. I'm going into week 6 and I love it. I am totally amazed with the difference it has made."

—Renee

"I'm a forty-six-year-old woman with ten children. Finding time has always been an issue for me, but your program is one that I have felt I could and must find the time to do. I now weigh a firm, toned 126 pounds and have the energy to keep up with everything that needs to be done around here, which is a lot!"

—Victoria

"Both my daughter (twenty-six years old) and I (fifty-two years old) have been on the program for about six months and have not only gained strength but also lost some weight. As we are both scientists, we were impressed that the information in the book was based on the results of published research and was presented in a sensible, rational manner."

—Nicola

"I am having such a good time with your strength-training program—I who have loathed exercise in all forms for all of my seventy-eight years. This is something I can do in the privacy of my home, with no huffing and puffing and running around. It makes me feel good and I quite look forward to my little sessions with the weights."

—Evelyn

"I was diagnosed with breast cancer in 1996 at the ripe old age of forty and I'm using your book to help me stay strong and healthy for whatever may come my way in the future."

—Kathy

"Five years ago I was very ill with chronic fatigue syndrome. I have slowly improved, but my muscles were very weak. When I first began your program I could not even lift one pound, so I worked without weights. Now, after a year, I am lifting nine pounds on the legs and four to ten pounds on the arm exercises. I am so thrilled and proud to be doing this!"

—Gaye

"I'm forty-eight years old. Before I began strength training, my arm would get tired when I washed my hair or even brushed my teeth. I was miserable, tired all the time, and just felt elderly. My doctor recommended your book, and I am amazed at what I can do after just three months."

—Jennifer

By the same authors

STRONG WOMEN STAY SLIM (Bantam)
STRONG WOMEN, STRONG BONES (Putnam)

CONTENTS

▼   ▼   ▼   ▼

IV: A LIFETIME OF FITNESS

In memory of
Elizabeth and Nanlee

▼   ▼   ▼   ▼

PREFACE

▼   ▼   ▼   ▼

Sports and physical activities have always been an important part of my life. As a child growing up in Pennsylvania, I skied, biked, swam, rode horses—whatever the season allowed. Knowing firsthand the benefits of being active, it was natural for me to choose a career that combined fitness and public health.

I was fortunate to do my graduate research at the Tufts University School of Nutrition. Scientists there were exploring the determinants of healthy aging, and I contributed to several early studies of the effects of exercise and nutrition on women's bone health. Outside the laboratory, I remained as active as ever—in fact, I completed three marathons while working toward my degree.

After receiving my doctorate, I was awarded a Congressional Research Fellowship and spent a year in the office of U.S. Senator Patrick Leahy from Vermont. This experience strengthened my desire to do research that would have an impact on public health. Though I thoroughly enjoyed my time in Washington, I missed the laboratory. So the following year I returned to Tufts and joined in the scientific efforts you will read about in this book.

Like other professionals in my field, I believe that exercise is essential to a healthy life. Many sedentary people want to change, but they don't have the accurate, practical information they need to get started. Filling this gap has become my personal mission. My research has proven that women can gain tremendous health benefits from simple strengthening exercises. These findings were published in the *Journal of the American Medical Association,* and I wanted them to reach the widest possible audience. The first edition of this book translated my research into a practical program that can be followed at home. Since its publication we've learned more about the benefits of strength training, and I've received responses and questions from thousands of readers. That's why I revised the book.

The greatest joy of my professional life is seeing women's lives change for the better as they become stronger. My own mother is one inspiring example. Though she wasn't particularly athletic when I was growing up, all that changed after she turned fifty. Now in her early seventies, she rides her mountain bike almost daily in the summer and cross-country skis in the winter. And convinced by my findings, she strength-trains year-round. Her energy and vibrancy are proof that strong women stay young.

ACKNOWLEDGMENTS

▼   ▼   ▼   ▼

This book, and the research on which it is based, would not have been possible without the help of many people. I want to thank these individuals and express my sincere respect and gratitude for all their assistance and support.

I am forever indebted to my mentors—three outstanding scientists who have guided my research and many other aspects of my professional life:

William J. Evans, Ph.D., with whom I have worked since 1983, has supported all my professional endeavors, always helping me to see the broader picture. He instilled in me the confidence that is so important to a young scientist. I'm also grateful to Bill for his careful review of this manuscript and his many helpful suggestions.

Maria A. Fiatarone, M.D., inspired me with her courageous research that shattered stereotypes about the physical limits of older people. My own work continues to follow her lead.

Irwin Rosenberg, M.D., energizes me with his excitement about science. Irv encourages me to listen to my heart, so I can focus on those topics I care most about.

I have learned so much from my other colleagues at Tufts and elsewhere. Particular thanks to Drs. Carmen Castaneda Sceppa, Christina Economos, Bess Dawson-Hughes, Roger Fielding, Walter Frontera, Jeanne Goldberg, Steven Heymsfield, James Judge, Christina Morganti, Richard

Pierson, Susan Roberts, and Ronenn Roubenoff. I am especially grateful to Roger Fielding for his careful review of the chapter on muscles, and to James Judge for his thoughtful comments on the balance chapter.

Brenda Crawford, O.T., Sharon Bortz, M.S., R.D., and Isaiah Trice, Ph.D., contributed enormously to my research with their technical and scientific support. Rarely do technicians receive the recognition they deserve—yet their dedication and their attention to detail ultimately are what make research successful.

I'm grateful to Robert N. Butler, M.D., and my colleagues at the Brookdale Foundation. The foundation provided not only financial support but also encouragement to translate my laboratory research into practical information for a broader audience.

The women who participated in my research deserve heartfelt thanks for their heroic efforts to better the lives of women. They journeyed regularly from their homes to the Tufts laboratory in downtown Boston. Their commitment was an inspiration. What I learned from them goes far beyond the findings of my study.

Writing a popular book was a new venture for me. Thanks to my colleagues in publishing, it has been a wonderful experience.

It is difficult to express the magnitude of thanks, admiration, and respect that I have for my collaborator, Sarah Wernick. Sarah approached me shortly after reading about my research and suggested I write a book to make it possible for all women to benefit from my findings. I am grateful for her amazing ability to make sense of my words and to capture the voices of women who have followed this program. She has become a dear friend.

Wendy Weil, my literary agent, was enthusiastic about this project right from the start. I feel so fortunate to have her support and expertise.

Toni Burbank, my editor, and her associates at Bantam have made the publishing process exciting and gratifying. Toni's critical guidance made the book much more readable and thorough—and at the same time she has been wonderfully supportive of my vision. I've appreciated the opportunity to participate in every stage as the manuscript was transformed into a book. The work doesn't stop there. I cherish the continuing support I've received from Robin Michaelson and Ryan Stellabotte, as well as the valuable efforts of Susan Corcoran, my publicist at Bantam.

Four wonderful writers—Anita Bartholemew, Sally Wendkos Olds, Pamela Painter, and Barbara Sofer—read early drafts of the manuscript. Their detailed comments greatly assisted me.

Wendy Wray did a wonderful job of translating exercises into beautiful and instructive illustrations. I appreciate her skill and her patience.

My Tufts colleagues provided invaluable help with the book.

Jennifer Layne, M.S., C.S.C.S., my research assistant, went above and beyond in her generous help. She worked with me on the exercises, discussed motivational issues, and even demonstrated the exercises for the illustrator. Her enthusiastic support has been a great inspiration, professionally and personally. Andrea Nuernberger, P.T., and Michael Wood, B.S., reviewed and brainstormed many of the exercises included in this book. Kristin Baker, Ph.D., assisted me with the muscle chapter. Melissa Bernstein, Ph.D., R.D., helped compile the nutrition information. Charles Pu, M.D., was willing to answer all my questions about medical aspects of the program. Rebecca Seguin, B.S., provided able assistance with research for the revised edition.

Special thanks to Larry Lindner and the *Tufts University Health & Nutrition Letter* for helping my research findings reach the general public.

For his review of the gym chapter, a warm thank-you to Dennis Keiser. His company has supported our research by donating strength-training machines to the Tufts laboratory, for which we are forever grateful.

I am indebted to Charlotte, Lisa, Maxine, Sarah, and Ursula, who tested the at-home version of the exercises week after week and offered very helpful comments. Working with them was one of the most enjoyable parts of this project. Special thanks as well to these research volunteers and others for sharing their personal observations: Andrea, Bea, Bernice, Bonnie, Dorothy, Evelyn, Flora, Jayne, Jean, Kathy, Laurie, Maida and her daughter Maida Lois, Mary Lou, Mimi, Miriam, Monica, Olive, Pat, Peg, Sara, Sherry, Susan, Thelma, Valerie, Verna, Al, John, and Sam.

Thank you to Leslie Abad, Coco McCabe, Lori Anderson, Robyn Wood, Katherine Edwards, and Mary Ann Hardenbergh who assisted with illustrations and various aspects of the book.

The steady, loving support of family and friends has made it possible for me to do my research and write this book. I especially want to thank my husband, Kin, and our children—Mason, Eliza, and Alexandra—for keeping me focused on the important things in life.

I

WHAT STRENGTH TRAINING WILL DO FOR YOU

YES, YOU CAN TURN
BACK THE CLOCK!

Ask Bernice for help, and she says, "Sure." Twice a week she chases after two young boys to give their mom a break. When her church needs a volunteer—whether it's to knit baby hats or to scramble eggs for a hundred people—they call Bernice. But she also finds time for herself. A few years ago she started an exercise program developed at Tufts University. A skeptical friend asked, "What are you trying to prove?" and Bernice retorted, "I don't want to feel old!" She credits the exercises for her excellent bowling scores and for her "great bursts of energy." Once, she took down all the first-floor curtains and washed them. While they were tumbling in the dryer, she cleaned the windows.

By the way, the boys are Bernice's great-grandchildren. Her bowling partners are in their seventies and eighties. Bernice herself is ninety-three—but definitely not old.

◆   ◆   ◆

Maida Lois used to stop her mother, also named Maida, when she started to lift something heavy. "Let me carry that for you," she'd say. "After all, I'm younger." The older Maida had never been physically active—until a few years ago, when she volunteered to be in an exercise study. At the end of the study, the two Maidas took a series of tests to compare their strength. At the time, the older Maida was sixty-six. Maida Lois was thirty-nine, and she trained for road races by running five miles five days a week. Maida Lois didn't hold back during the tests. "I got competitive," she admits; "I tried hard."

It didn't help. Maida outscored her daughter by 12 to 18 percent on three of the four strength tests and was only 8 percent behind on the fourth. After that, Maida did her own lifting. "After all," she'd tell Maida Lois, "I'm stronger."

◆   ◆   ◆

Even in high school, Evelyn wore a size 16. At age thirty, she had her first child, and her weight climbed to over 200 pounds. Soon afterward, she came to work at Tufts University. "I became interested in nutrition, I started doing aerobics, and I got down to 160 pounds. I was thinner, but I was complete flab," she recalls. What's more, her weight loss had reached a plateau. Inspired by her colleagues' research—and the success stories all around her—Evelyn started an exercise program. "It toned my body and speeded up my metabolism. I took off the last thirty pounds."

Now thirty-eight and the mother of two, Evelyn recently attended her twentieth high school reunion. She describes a thrilling evening: "Some of my best girlfriends never got back in shape after having kids—and there I was in a slinky black evening dress, size 6. I got compliments from men who never spoke to me in high school."

◆   ◆   ◆

As one of the scientists who developed these remarkably successful exercise programs, I'm very proud of Bernice, Maida, and Evelyn. They were willing to try something that was not only challenging but unusual for women: high-intensity strength training. Our studies have proven that the benefits they gained were not unique. If you're a woman age thirty-five or older, you should know what strength training can do for you.

Let me tell you about my part in this research. For my study, I recruited forty postmenopausal women. All were healthy but sedentary; none was taking hormones. Half the volunteers—our control group—were simply asked to maintain their usual lifestyle for the next year. Their before-and-after measurements would show us what physical changes a woman can expect after a year just because she's that much older. The others—including Maida—came twice a week to our laboratory and lifted weights.

Most women begin to lose bone and muscle mass at about age forty; in part because of this, they start to slow down. And that's exactly what happened to the women who didn't exercise. One sedentary year later, their muscles and bones had aged and they were even less active than before.

The women who lifted weights changed too—but in the opposite direction. **After one year of strength training, their bodies were fifteen to twenty years more youthful.**

Instead of losing bone density, they actually showed small but significant *gains.* Their scores on strength tests soared to levels more typical of women in their late thirties or early forties. All the participants had agreed not to gain or lose weight, because that might have confused our results. But those in the strength-training group traded fat for muscle. So they looked trimmer—and some even dropped a dress size or two.

As these physical changes unfolded, we saw emotional changes too. The women felt happier, more energetic, more self-confident. Self-imposed stereotypes shattered, and their lives began to change.

One surprise was that our volunteers became much more active as they got stronger. We had specifically asked them not to join any fitness programs during the year—a routine precaution to make sure other factors weren't responsible for the changes we were measuring. But on their twice-weekly visits, they described other ventures:

- ♦ Sheila, fifty-eight, announced, "I went Rollerblading with my husband last weekend!"
- ♦ Nancy, fifty-three, reported: "My husband and I took our first canoe trip in years. We'd stopped because I couldn't help him get the canoe on the car—and now I can."

- ♦ Flora, sixty-six, who previously brushed off a friend's invitations to go ballroom dancing, finally tried it. She had such a good time, she started dancing several evenings a week.
- ♦ Verna, sixty-eight, moved four tons of topsoil that a dump truck deposited in her driveway. The pile was taller than Verna, wider than a car. As incredulous neighbors watched, she tackled the dirt with a shovel and a wheelbarrow. "I worked three hours a day, then four," Verna told us. "I never had any aches or pains." A week later, the driveway was clear and the topsoil was in the garden.

At the end of the year, the women who strength-trained not only felt younger but were leading more youthful lives. What's more, the changes have continued. Since she completed her year with us, Maida—once sedentary—has developed a whole new lifestyle. She works out at a gym three or four times a week. In the winter, she ice skates; in the summer, she switches to in-line skates or rides her six-speed bike—a birthday gift from her three children. And year-round there's line dancing two nights a week. She says: "I'm in better health now than I've ever been in my whole life. I have more confidence in attempting physical things. I never think about age."

A few summers ago Maida joined her daughter and a group of Maida Lois's friends for a demanding raft trip through the Grand Canyon. Maida Lois says:

> Before the trip, my mother kept asking, "Do you think they'll mind taking an old lady along?" But everyone thought she was amazing. There were many side hikes—two- or three-hour climbs up to side canyons and waterfalls—and she did all of them. We had the best time. She's in better shape than any of her contemporaries. I know she's nearly seventy, but she looks more in her fifties. I don't think of her as old in any way.

Inspired by Maida's example—and that mother-daughter testing session—Maida Lois started strength training herself. Though she was physically active before, lifting weights has made a difference. She says:

I have a lot more energy than I had when I was just running. My job is demanding. By mid-afternoon I used to need a cup of strong coffee to make it through the rest of the day. Now I don't. I'm not as stressed. I feel better about myself across the board.

Our volunteers turned back the clock with just two strength-training sessions a week. They recovered bone; they recovered muscle. But even more important, they recovered energy and enjoyment of life they thought they had lost forever.

These dramatic findings may sound too good to be true, but I can assure you they're not. This study was conducted at the world-renowned Jean Mayer USDA Human Nutrition Research Center on Aging at Tufts University. Our report was scrutinized carefully by other scientists and accepted for publication by the *Journal of the American Medical Association (JAMA)*—one of the most prestigious medical journals in the world.

When the study appeared in December 1994, it drew an outpouring of interest. Dozens of newspaper and magazine articles were written about our work; I was interviewed on many TV and radio programs. I received hundreds of queries asking: "Please tell me how to do those exercises!" That is why I wrote *Strong Women Stay Young.*

After this book was first published in 1997, thousands of women, fitness professionals, and doctors contacted me. Their feedback helped me refine the exercise program, making it easier and more efficient. I developed instructions for men in response to requests from physicians, male readers—and my own father and husband. Meanwhile, scientific findings continued to accumulate, documenting the benefits of strength training. I decided to revise *Strong Women Stay Young* so I could incorporate all these improvements and new information.

IS THIS BOOK FOR YOU?

Let me ask you some pointed questions:

- ◆ Have you lost strength over the past decade?
- ◆ Do you ever say, "I know I should exercise, but I just don't have the energy"?

- At the end of a normally busy day, do you feel tired and worn out?
- Do you notice fat where there used to be muscle?
- Do you feel older than you'd like?
- Is it more difficult to maintain your weight—even though you're eating less?
- Are your favorite sports harder and less fun than they used to be?
- Do you look at your older female relatives and worry that someday you'll be just as limited physically as they are now?

For many women past thirty-five, these changes—the loss of strength, the lack of vigor—are painfully familiar. If you're experiencing them, you may have figured it's all an inevitable part of getting older. Wrong! Scientists at Tufts and elsewhere now know this isn't true. The main reason most people slow down when they get older is that they lose about a third of their muscle mass between ages thirty-five and eighty. Yes, aging plays a role. However, inactivity is a major factor—and that's something you can address.

If you've ever been bedridden for a few days and felt weak when you tried to get up again, you know what inactivity does to your body. A sedentary lifestyle doesn't take its toll quite so rapidly, but it inflicts the same damage. The first signs are subtle: Your legs tire more quickly during a brisk walk; briefcases and grocery bags seem heavier. You need to rest in the middle of a museum visit. After a few decades, even such simple acts as standing up from a low sofa may become difficult.

My mentor, Irwin Rosenberg, M.D., director of the Tufts Center on Aging, coined a word for this transformation: *sarcopenia,* from the Greek *sarco* for "flesh" or "muscle," and *penia* for "loss." Unlike heart disease and cancer, sarcopenia doesn't actually kill. But more than any other single factor, muscle loss is responsible for the frailty and diminished vitality we associate with old age.

This doesn't have to happen to you! Our research has shown that sarcopenia can be prevented to a very great extent—and if the process has begun, it can be reversed.

If you've lost strength, you can regain it.

If your energy has sagged, you can raise it.

If you've lost muscle and gained fat, you can reverse it.

If you've become flabby, you can get trim.

If you feel older than you like, you can feel younger, stronger, and more vigorous—perhaps better than you've ever felt in your entire life.

**Strength training, we have learned,
is a fountain of youth.**

WHAT'S NEW IN THE REVISED EDITION?

If you read the original *Strong Women Stay Young,* you may be wondering how this version is different. Here's what's new:

- ♦ Updated scientific information about muscle, bone, and balance
- ♦ Streamlined basic workout that takes 30 minutes instead of 40, with two new moves and three updated exercises
- ♦ Six supplemental exercises, nearly all new or revamped
- ♦ Workouts that strengthen the back, tone the abs, and relieve achy shoulders, plus step-by-step instructions for creating customized strengthening routines that go beyond the basics
- ♦ Expanded resource lists for additional information about nutrition and exercise
- ♦ A chapter with instructions for men

If you've been following the program in the original *Strong Women Stay Young* or in *Strong Women Stay Slim,* you can keep doing the same exercises. But now you have additional options. Use the instructions on page 202 to mix and match.

PIONEERING RESEARCH ON STRENGTH TRAINING

I first came to the Tufts Center on Aging in 1983, when I was a graduate student. At the time, our research focused on the effects of aerobic activity. Then, in the mid-1980s, one of our scientists, Walter Frontera, M.D., under the direction of the center's physiology laboratory chief, William Evans, Ph.D., decided to look at a different kind of exercise: strength training. And they decided to work the volunteers—men in their sixties and seventies—at a higher intensity than any researchers had ever done before.

At the time, scientists generally believed that loss of muscle and strength were inevitable as people got older and that neither could be restored. The few previous studies of strength training in this age group had measured the maximum subjects could lift, then put them on a program using weights that were only about half as heavy. Anything more, the investigators assumed, might cause injuries or cardiac problems. These timid programs didn't accomplish much—in strength training, feeble efforts produce puny results.

Not discouraged by conventional wisdom, Dr. Frontera took a different approach. Younger athletes trained with weights almost as heavy as their maximum, because low-intensity workouts didn't make them stronger. Why, he wondered, would older people be any different? Instead of working out at 40 to 50 percent of their capacity, his volunteers exercised at 80 percent.

The findings shattered myths about aging. There were no injuries, no cardiac episodes. These men didn't merely survive a challenging strength-training program, they thrived. In just twelve weeks, the muscles they were exercising became 10 to 12 percent larger and a whopping 100 to 175 percent stronger. Most of the men reported with delight that they were now stronger than ever before.

These results inspired an even more startling research proposal from a new member of our group, Maria Fiatarone, M.D. If strength training could help sixty-year-olds, she reasoned, it should be even more beneficial for the very weakest men and women—the frail elderly.

Together with William Evans, Dr. Fiatarone approached the medical director of a nursing home, asking permission to conduct a small strength-training study with volunteer residents. They had a lot of explaining to do. No, this wasn't one of those typical exercise programs for the elderly, where they sat, extended their arms, and slowly made circles in the air. These research subjects would be doing high-intensity strengthening workouts on the same kind of machines twenty-five-year-olds use at the gym.

The medical director was skeptical, to say the least. How could it possibly be safe for a nursing home resident to lift weights? But Drs. Fiatarone and Evans convincingly explained the logic of the program, which was based on principles of rehabilitation medicine: Start at a safe level and progress gradually as strength increases.

You can hardly imagine a less likely group for an exercise study than the six women and four men who volunteered to work out with Dr. Fiatarone. They ranged in age from eighty-six to ninety-six. Some people remain vigorous in their nineties, but these were typical nursing home residents. All had at least two serious chronic diseases, including heart disease, diabetes, and osteoporosis. Most relied on walkers or canes, and several had leg muscles so weak they couldn't rise from a chair without assistance from their arms. But three times a week, for eight weeks, they faithfully came to the exercise room at the nursing home and they lifted weights.

The results—published in *JAMA* in 1990—were truly remarkable. In just eight weeks, these frail elderly men and women increased their strength by an average 175 percent. On a test of walking speed and balance, their scores rose by an average of 48 percent. Two participants discarded their canes. These findings inspired larger clinical trials in our lab and elsewhere—and all confirmed the benefits of strength training.

Meanwhile, I had been studying women ages fifty to seventy, looking in particular at the effects of walking and other aerobic exercise on bone. As findings accumulated about strength training—including animal studies that suggested it could increase bone density—I began to wonder if strengthening exercises could help women's bones too. Together with Drs. Fiatarone and Evans, I designed a study to investigate this question. The results were even more exciting than expected.

WHAT STRENGTH TRAINING CAN DO FOR YOU

We now know that a challenging, progressive strength-training program can build muscles and increase strength in men and women of all ages. But my study proved that the benefits go even further. Besides the great gains in strength, here's what strength training does:

♦ HALTS BONE LOSS—AND EVEN RESTORES BONE

Each year after menopause, a woman typically loses 1 percent of her bone mass—even more during the first five postmenopausal years. Over time, she may develop *osteoporosis,* a condition in which bones become so porous they easily break. Strength training stopped the clock here too. The women who didn't exercise lost about 2 percent of their bone density over the year of the study. But the women who strength-trained not only didn't lose bone, they *gained* 1 percent.

♦ IMPROVES BALANCE

Our ability to stay in balance also declines with passing years. The change happens so slowly we may not notice it until we're in our seventies. But falling—the result of deteriorated balance—becomes a significant hazard later in life, especially if bones are weak. The women who didn't exercise showed an 8.5 percent decline in balance over the study period. In contrast, the women in the strength-training group improved their balancing ability—their test scores went up by 14 percent.

♦ HELPS PREVENT BONE FRACTURES FROM OSTEOPOROSIS

The improvements in strength, bone density, and balance have special significance for women because they dramatically reduce the risk of fractures from osteoporosis. This is a serious problem for older women: A woman of seventy faces 30 percent odds that she will break her hip if she lives another twenty years.

Hormones, calcium supplements, and medications offer significant protection from bone loss. However, strength training not only builds bone, it cuts the risk of fractures by improving strength and balance to help prevent falls. What's more, all these benefits come without worrisome side effects.

♦ ENERGIZES

At the beginning and end of the study, we asked our volunteers how much they walked, how many stairs they climbed, and how much time they spent on energetic recreational activities. When we added it all up, the nonexercise group had become 25 percent less active. But the women in the strength-training program were *27 percent more active* than before. It makes sense: The stronger you are, the easier it is to move.

This is an exciting finding because an active lifestyle has far-reaching health benefits. As underscored by the 1996 Surgeon General's Report, physical activity helps decrease disease and disability, improves mental health, and actually increases longevity. I now encourage sedentary women to begin strength training *before* they attempt aerobics. If their muscles are weak, aerobic exercise will be difficult. But after a month or two of strength training, they often find that an aerobic workout has become fun.

♦ TRIMS AND TIGHTENS

Weight loss and body shaping weren't goals of the study we reported in *JAMA*—remember, we asked participants to maintain their weight over the year. Though the scale didn't change, their appearance did. Instead of dropping *pounds*, the women who exercised lost *inches*.

♦ HELPS CONTROL WEIGHT

Gaining muscle not only promotes aerobic activity, which burns calories, but also boosts metabolism. That's because muscle is active tissue and consumes calories; stored fat, on the other hand, is inert and uses very little energy. As I explain in my second book, *Strong Women Stay Slim,* dieters often lose muscle along with fat. We found, in a small preliminary study, that women who strength-trained while following a weight-reduction program maintained muscle as the pounds melted away. Pat, seventy-six,

one of the volunteers in this study, lost twenty-nine pounds—all of it fat—
and has kept most of it off for four and a half years. She comments:

> *I burn 160 more calories per day just because my metabolism is
> higher. You know how after you go off a diet you want to eat
> everything in sight, especially the things you haven't been eating?
> When you get rid of the fat and have more muscle, then you can
> eat a little more and not feel deprived.*

◆ Improves Flexibility

Though this wasn't a focus of my *JAMA* study, women kept telling
me that strength training had made them more flexible. Pat says:

> *I used to struggle to fasten that tiny button in back of my silk
> blouse, and my arm would hurt a little. Now I do it without
> thinking about it.*

◆ Revitalizes

The *JAMA* report focused on muscles, bones, and balance. But as far
as I'm concerned, the most exciting part of this study was something harder
to measure: the transformation of our volunteers. They didn't expect their
bodies could change much, not at their age. But after just a few months they
were stronger, trimmer, and more energetic than they ever dreamed they
could be again—and they were thrilled. Who wouldn't be?

◆ A Health Tonic?

The more we look at strength training, the more benefits we find. Recent studies at Tufts and elsewhere suggest that strength training reduces the
risk of heart disease and adult-onset diabetes, lifts depression and boosts
self-esteem, eases sleep problems, relieves symptoms of both rheumatoid
and osteoarthritis, combats constipation and stress incontinence—and even
improves the quality of life for people with AIDS. I'm confident you'll be
hearing more about strength training in the future. So watch for news of the
latest developments.

MYTHS ABOUT
STRENGTH TRAINING

Many women—particularly those who have never been physically active—are skeptical when I tell them they'll benefit from strength training. Some fear they're incapable of following this program; they assume it's too late for them to get strong. Others, who are already physically active, believe they're doing enough. Don't let these five common myths hold you back.

Myth 1: "I don't need strength training because I do aerobics."

Aerobic exercise is essential for cardiovascular fitness, and it has many other important health benefits. But it won't make you strong. I've seen marathon runners with trim, muscular legs, but flabby, underdeveloped upper bodies and arms. Nor will you become strong from walking—though, of course, it's a fantastic exercise for your heart. The ultimate irony, if you're trying to stay fit, would be to live to old age with a healthy heart—only to find yourself too feeble to remain independent.

I'm definitely *not* suggesting that you abandon your current fitness regimen, just recommending that you make strength training a part of it. In fact, most elite endurance athletes do exactly that to improve their performance and prevent injuries. If you aren't already doing aerobic exercise, this program can help you start—when your muscles are prepared, aerobic workouts are much more enjoyable.

Myth 2: "Lifting weights will make me look muscle-bound and masculine."

Many people confuse strength training with body building, which aims for bulk. But strength training has long been Hollywood's secret for staying slim. Only recently did we learn that Marilyn Monroe kept her curvaceous body in shape by lifting weights. Women bodybuilders go to great lengths to produce those bulky muscles. They use extremely heavy weights, have lengthy workouts, and often take steroids and follow rigorous diets. This program doesn't approach those extremes of effort or results.

The women in my *JAMA* study wound up *smaller,* not larger. Their muscles increased by an average of 9 percent, enough to make an enormous difference in their strength. But they lost a corresponding amount of fat—and since muscle is denser than fat, they were trimmer. No one complained about looking unfeminine. On the contrary, they were delighted with their slimmer figures.

Myth 3: "I can't afford to join a gym or buy costly equipment."

You can follow this program at home using readily available hand and leg weights that cost under $150—much less than a treadmill or other fancy machines. Some women reduce the price tag even further by sharing equipment or by purchasing used weights. Those who prefer to train on machines don't necessarily have to join an expensive gym. Many have access to strength-training equipment at work or at a Y or community center.

Myth 4: "I'm so out of shape that I'd hurt myself if I tried to lift weights."

If ninety-year-old nursing home residents can do strength training, chances are that you can too. Under medical supervision, strengthening exercises are appropriate for men and women with heart disease, as well as for those who suffer from arthritis, osteoporosis, and other chronic but stable medical conditions. In fact, the weaker you are, the more you need this program! You'll work out at a level that's appropriate for you; as you get stronger, the program adapts to your new abilities.

What's risky is *not* exercising. In my *JAMA* study, the women who strength-trained had no serious injuries. But those who continued their usual sedentary lives were not so lucky. Two of these women broke their wrists. One was Bonnie, who recalls:

I'd been disappointed not to be in the exercise group, because I was very interested in doing weight lifting. Then I had a very bad wrist break, and strength training was part of my rehabilitation. That was in 1992. I still work out three times a week. If I'm away and can't do it, I miss it.

Myth 5: "I'm in my forties—a program for older women won't do anything for me."

I follow this program—and I'm a former competitive endurance athlete in my thirties who's still very active! Indeed, so do many of my male colleagues and friends. Strength-training principles are the same regardless of your age or sex. It's really very simple: You work out with a weight that's just heavy enough so you can lift it eight times in good form before you have to rest. As you get stronger, and that weight is no longer challenging enough, you increase the load.

True, most men and younger women can start this program with heavier weights than most ninety-year-olds; also, they typically wind up being stronger. But that's really the only difference. The moves are the same and the instructions for progressing are the same.

HOW THIS BOOK WILL HELP YOU

The *Strong Women Stay Young* program goes far beyond the five exercises I used for my *JAMA* study. Those exercises were performed using sophisticated machines and were designed to provide scientific information. For this book, I wanted to create an at-home program for all women—not just those with access to a modern gym. Most of all, I wanted you to have the best possible all-around program, based on up-to-the-minute information. Because some women might prefer to train at a gym, I've included a chapter with instructions for a strength-training program using machines.

Here's what you will get from this book:

◆ A Practical Program Even a Couch Potato Can Do

The exercises are simple—even simpler overall than the original *SWSY* program. Unlike aerobics, they're literally no-sweat. There's no need to get down on the floor (and struggle up again), because everything is done standing or seated on a chair. And you don't need a Lycra leotard or any other special clothes.

The program doesn't take a lot of time. You can exercise at home, with just two thirty-minute sessions per week: one in front of the evening news and the other during the Saturday night movie.

Results are rapid. You will see significant improvements in just four weeks.

◆ A Program Challenging Enough for Active Women

This book will be helpful even if you've done strength training before. Unless you received accurate information, you may not be getting the full benefit you deserve for your efforts. For instance, many women, misled by popular advice, faithfully lift soup cans in the hope of improving their muscles. Or they work out with three-pound weights week after week in a "Tone and Firm" class. Sadly, these approaches don't make you stronger. Weights must be considerably heavier than soup cans to make a difference. And if you don't systematically increase the load as your muscles develop, you won't progress very far.

◆ Medically Proven Exercises and Training Principles

You can rely on the safety and effectiveness of this program. It's based on scientifically tested programs developed at Tufts University. Those, in turn, drew upon long-established principles from physical rehabilitation medicine. Indeed, if you've worked with a physical therapist, you may recognize some of the exercises.

Before you begin, you'll answer a few simple strength-assessment questions to determine a safe starting point. As you grow stronger, you'll add weights. No matter how fit you are now, no matter how quickly or slowly you progress, **the program will always be right for you.**

◆ Up-to-the-Minute Scientific Information

If you can't wait to start, you can jump ahead to Part II. But most people find they're even more motivated if they understand not only *how* to do the exercises but *why* they work. So I've included three chapters with the latest information:

- ◆ Chapter 2 explains how our muscles work; why they stop working if they're not used—and how to wake them up again.
- ◆ Chapter 3 takes a look at bone, which can silently slip away as we get older—unless we do something about it.
- ◆ Chapter 4 discusses balance, our remarkable ability to remain upright—which should never be taken for granted.

◆ Step-by-Step Instructions

This book gives you a complete program, customized to your level of fitness.

- ◆ Chapter 6 takes you shopping for equipment.
- ◆ Chapter 7 provides strength-training basics—everything from a readiness test to safety cautions for your back.
- ◆ Chapter 8 is the heart of the *Strong Women Stay Young* program: eight simple exercises that will make you stronger.
- ◆ Chapter 9 explains how to customize the program—where to start, how to progress, and what to aim for.
- ◆ Chapter 13 has information about the benefits of strength training for men, along with directions they can use to follow the program in this book.

◆ ATTENTION TO MOTIVATION

No exercise program works if it's not followed. We work hard at motivating our participants—and it pays off. *The dropout rates in our studies are as low as in any exercise research reported in the medical literature.*

I consider motivation so important that I've devoted two chapters to the subject:

- Chapter 5 reveals how to move from *thinking* about the program to *doing* it.
- Chapter 10 tells you everything we've discovered about how to keep yourself on track.

◆ OPTIONS FOR THE FUTURE

Strength training will make remarkable changes in your body after just a few weeks. But if it doesn't become a lifelong habit, the benefits will be lost. To help you continue, I've suggested ways to vary the program:

- Chapter 11 presents six additional strengthening exercises, with instructions for creating a variety of new workouts— from a routine that tightens your abs to a mini-program done without weights that you can follow when you're away from home.
- Chapter 12 provides a complete program for strength training at a gym, plus tips on selecting a facility or trainer.

You're about to start a program that will improve the quality of your life—not just now but for years to come. It's an exciting program because progress is so rapid and so visible. As you become stronger, everything you do will become easier. Like many women, you may find this applies to more than physical activities. Strength training challenges your muscles. But it also dares you to venture beyond limiting stereotypes and to develop in unexpected ways. As your muscles grow, so will your self-confidence and self-esteem.

EMPOWERING
YOUR MUSCLES

◆ ◆ ◆

I went to a track meet at my granddaughter's high school, and I was amazed to see girls competing while their boyfriends cheered them on. When I was that age, a girl was considered odd if she did anything like that. One time I ran to get the school bus and when I got on, the guys were whooping and hollering. I asked a friend why they were laughing, and she said, "It's you. Don't do that, or they won't ask you out." I think it's great that women today can do anything they want to.

  —Pat

Strength training is a great conversation starter. When people ask me what's new, I tell them I'm lifting weights. After they fall down and look at me as if I'm out of my mind, I explain. I get totally positive feedback. My daughter and her college friends call me Power Woman.

  —Lisa

◆ ◆ ◆

Y ou may not think of yourself as muscular, but you are. Your body contains more than six hundred muscles, and together they account for a third to a half of your weight. Muscles power your every move, whether it's the swing of a tennis racket or the blink of an eye. They also make your heart beat, push air in and out of your lungs, and perform dozens of other vital functions.

As children and young adults, women have all the muscular capacity they need. But midlife brings changes. Starting at around age forty, most women lose nearly half a pound of muscle each year and gain the same amount of fat—until, by age eighty, they have only a third of the muscle mass they had at forty. This is the transformation called **sarcopenia.**

Muscle loss was once thought to be an inevitable part of aging. When older patients complained about weakness and reduced stamina, doctors used to say, "What do you expect, at your age? Get used to it." Today, for the first time, we can offer a much better solution: strength training. Our research has proven that strengthening exercise not only delays sarcopenia for decades but actually *reverses* the process. What's more, when we boost the amount of muscle in our bodies, the benefits go beyond strength.

"USE IT OR LOSE IT"

T he first astronauts entered their space capsules in top-notch physical condition—and returned from their missions as weak as if they'd been lying in bed the whole time. How come? Because they were weightless in space, they didn't need their muscles to move around. The effect was remarkable: In just a few days, these healthy, vigorous men lost significant amounts of muscle and strength. NASA scientists moved quickly to correct the problem, and today's astronauts exercise on machines to help keep their muscles in shape.

The same principle applies to age-related muscle loss. Men and women who work their muscles retain significantly more strength as they get older. And even those who belatedly adopt a more healthful lifestyle can regain previously lost muscle mass and ward off sarcopenia.

A

Strength training can make your thighs young again.

These are CAT scans showing the cross sections of thighs. The innermost white portion with the dark center is bone and bone marrow. The lighter gray is muscle, and the layer around the muscle is fat.

Picture A shows the thigh of a moderately active twenty-five-year-old woman.

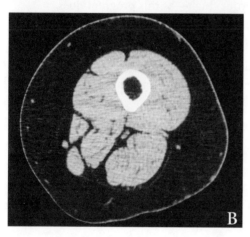

B

Picture B shows the thigh of a sedentary fifty-eight-year-old woman. The older woman has much more fat, much less muscle. But the chief culprit is inactivity, not age. Take a look at picture C.

C

This thigh is similar to the youthful one in picture A, but it belongs to a woman who completed my strength-training study—and she's sixty-three years old!

MUSCLE BASICS

I f you know what's going on behind the scenes, you'll understand how strength training affects you. Look at the drawing of your **skeletal muscles**—the muscles that move your body. Skeletal muscles are attached to your bones, either directly or by tendons.

While one muscle works, others perform complementary actions to keep your bones aligned. For instance, if your biceps (the muscle in front of your upper arm) lifts a dumbbell, your triceps (the muscle in back of your upper arm) stabilizes your elbow. That's why it's important to train certain muscles in pairs—the biceps and the triceps; the quadriceps and the hamstrings in the front and back of your thigh—as this program does.

Your muscles perform three basic types of actions.

1. **Concentric:** the muscle gets shorter. When you pick up a dumbbell, the biceps shortens to bring your forearm up.

2. **Eccentric:** the muscle lengthens. When you slowly lower the dumbbell, your biceps is performing an eccentric action.

3. **Isometric** (also called *static*): the muscle exerts force, but its length remains the same. An example is holding the dumbbell up, with your biceps supporting the weight but not moving it.

Eccentric actions stimulate the most muscle development. That's why I'll remind you to lower weights slowly—if you let gravity do the work, your muscles will miss out on the eccentric part of the move. It's also important to avoid the other extreme, subjecting your muscles to excessive eccentric effort. We've studied the consequences, using exercises that involve only eccentric action, such as lowering weights. Though these workouts don't seem too strenuous at the time, one to two days later volunteers feel very sore; their muscles are inflamed. Sometimes they even develop a fever and mild flulike symptoms. If you've ever experienced delayed soreness a day after a long, steep descent on a hike, it's because walking downhill involves eccentric muscle action.

The exercises in this book will *not* cause these extremely unpleasant

Skeletal Muscles

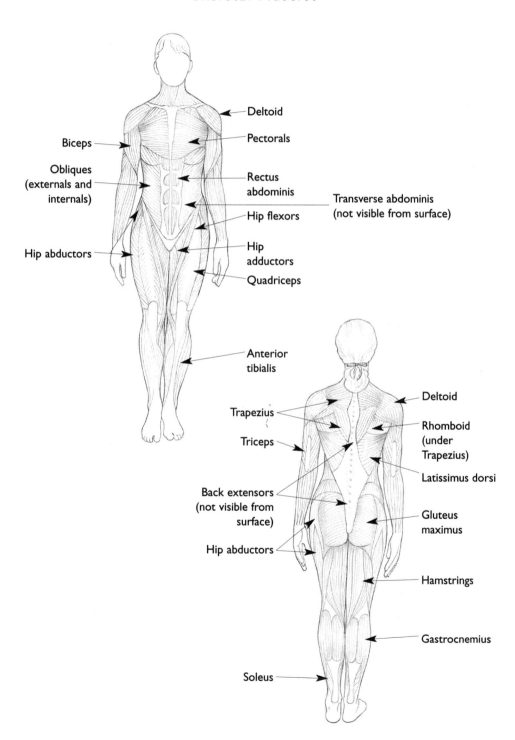

Deltoid

Biceps

Pectorals

Obliques
(externals and
internals)

Rectus
abdominis

Transverse abdominis
(not visible from surface)

Hip flexors

Hip abductors

Hip
adductors

Quadriceps

Anterior
tibialis

Deltoid

Trapezius

Rhomboid
(under
Trapezius)

Triceps

Latissimus dorsi

Back extensors
(not visible from
surface)

Gluteus
maximus

Hip abductors

Hamstrings

Gastrocnemius

Soleus

OTHER MUSCLES

Skeletal muscles are not the only kind you have.

Your heart consists almost entirely of **cardiac muscle,** which is found nowhere else in the body. Aerobic exercise—a workout that increases your heart rate—is the best way to keep cardiac muscle strong. Though strength training is not aerobic, it can improve aerobic capacity, especially if you're out of shape.

Smooth muscle is found in your internal organs and the walls of your blood vessels. These muscles perform many different tasks, from dilating and contracting the irises of your eyes to moving food through your digestive tract. They even help regulate body temperature—your blood vessels dilate to give off heat and constrict to conserve heat. Though we can't train smooth muscles directly, we know that aerobic exercise improves their performance. Preliminary studies suggest that strength training may produce similar effects.

effects! First, every exercise includes both concentric and eccentric components. Second, the weight you lift will match your concentric strength, which is less than your eccentric strength. Indeed, you'll tap only about half of your eccentric strength when you train at the proper intensity.

◆ ◆ ◆

My lying age is twenty-six, but I was seventy when I did the Tufts study. I always felt that lifting weights was something young, vigorous people do. I had visions of things cracking and crumbling. But nothing cracked and nothing crumbled.
—Pat

◆ ◆ ◆

THE IMPACT OF STRENGTH TRAINING

Let's trace what happens when you lift a dumbbell. This simple move starts with a nerve impulse, a signal from your brain. The impulse runs down your spinal cord, then it branches to nerves in your arm and speeds toward your biceps.

Like all muscles, the biceps is made up of tiny threadlike tissues called **myofibrils** that are bundled together into **muscle fibers.** Groups of muscle fibers are clustered into **motor units,** all under the control of a single nerve.

When the nerve impulse arrives at a biceps motor unit, it releases a **neurotransmitter**—a chemical that acts like a mini-jolt of electricity—and makes your muscle fibers contract for a fraction of a second. This is called **firing the muscle.** When you bend your elbow, it feels as if the muscle is contracting just once. But, in fact, it's firing 50 to 150 times, repeatedly contracting and relaxing like the unseen flicker of a fluorescent light that appears to be glowing steadily. Indeed, if something goes wrong, and your muscle fibers contract continuously, you feel a cramp.

Like the rest of your body, muscles get their fuel from the food you eat, which is digested and distributed via the bloodstream. This is not a simple process! Complex biochemical factors affect how much nourishment is released to your muscles and how it's metabolized.

When you begin a challenging strength-training program, such as the one in this book, *every part* of this process improves. So don't be surprised if you experience seemingly unrelated benefits. Here's what strength training does:

◆ SENDS A WAKE-UP CALL TO YOUR NERVES

Almost immediately, strength training reactivates motor units that have become dormant because of inactivity. Exercise also seems to teach the motor units to coordinate their firing more successfully. Imagine six people standing around a heavy banquet table trying to lift it. If they didn't cooperate, the table wouldn't budge. But if everyone lifted at exactly the same moment, the table would rise.

Strength training also affects the **inhibitory reflex**—a protective reflex that prevents our muscles from contracting so hard that they damage bones and connective tissues. Training partly suppresses the reflex, so our muscles have freer rein. By the way, scientists speculate that the same reflex is suppressed in extreme situations; this could explain those seemingly superhuman feats of strength we sometimes read about in the tabloids—such as a mother saving her child's life after an auto accident by lifting the car.

♦ STIMULATES MUSCLE CELL GROWTH

Muscle cells atrophy if they aren't used. Strength training does the opposite: It causes muscle to **hypertrophy**—that is, enlarge. We believe this growth is stimulated by microstructural "damage," harmless changes in the muscle that you couldn't see without a microscope. This is just a revved-up version of the normal breaking down and repair of cells from the wear and tear of everyday life.

Hypertrophy sounds scary, but don't worry: This program makes muscles a lot stronger but only slightly larger. For instance, after a year of strength training, the thighs of the women in our *JAMA* study averaged 73 percent stronger. But their thigh muscles were only 8 percent bigger—not a difference you'd notice. And in most cases, loss of fat more than compensated for the gain.

♦ BOOSTS HELPFUL ENZYMES

When muscles grow and become more active, our bodies increase production of various beneficial enzymes. Some help the muscles store and use fuel; others aid in waste disposal. What's particularly interesting about this change is that it seems to affect *all* your muscles, not just the ones you're training.

CAN STRENGTH TRAINING RELIEVE URINARY STRESS INCONTINENCE?

I wanted to share an unexpected benefit of your program. I was fairly active when I started. But I used to suffer stress incontinence, especially when I was running or playing tennis. It was putting a damper on my fitness program! Now I find this is much improved. I'm delighted—I was starting to wear incontinence pads when I went running.
—Kathy

Stress incontinence—leaking of urine under "stresses" like sneezing, laughing, or exercising—is a common problem in women. I don't know of any scientific study showing that strength training helps, but Kathy is not the first woman to tell me she's experienced an improvement. The exercises in the *Strong Women* program might not seem relevant since they work the arms and legs. But strength training has beneficial effects on body chemistry that make all muscles function better. So it really isn't surprising that the muscles that control urine flow would be stronger too.

If you suffer from urinary stress incontinence, ask your health care provider about the Kegel exercises, which address those muscles directly. It's very helpful to have feedback when you're learning them, something readily done during a vaginal exam.

Or have a look at the website of the Iowa Women's Health Center, which provides detailed instructions for the Kegel exercises: http://obgyn.uihc.uiowa.edu/Patinfo/urogyn/kegel.htm

WHEN TO EXPECT RESULTS

This program is exciting because you progress very quickly. Within two months, women in our studies typically *double* the amount of weight they can lift! That's because strength training reactivates motor nerves right away. By the eighth week, nerve improvements start to slow down. From this point on, gains in strength come primarily from the muscles themselves.

The following chart shows how the women in my *JAMA* study progressed over the year. About half of their strength gains came in the first three months, and about three-quarters came by the end of six months. Later gains were smaller and slower. However, even after a year, these women were still getting stronger. Would they have reached a limit eventually? We can't be sure. A Canadian investigator, who followed a group of elderly men and women for two years, found no end to the improvements.

◆ ◆ ◆

My upper arms feel different. When I was in the shower, I noticed a rounding and there was a hardness there again. It took me by surprise—I've been doing the program for just a month and I never thought I would see anything so quickly.
—Ursula

◆ ◆ ◆

MORE MUSCLE MEANS LESS FAT

As I've explained, the women in my *JAMA* study had agreed to maintain their starting body weight—the point was to let us focus on the effects of the exercise program without having to take other factors into account. Even though the scale didn't budge, the women became *leaner:* their bodies had less fat and more muscle. As a result they lost inches. Dorothy wore a size 16 when she joined our program. After just six months of strength training, she needed a new wardrobe:

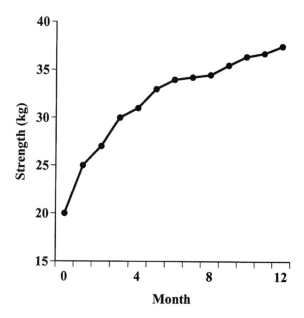

This shows how women in my *JAMA* study increased their strength in the knee extension exercise, which is also part of the program in this book. The pattern of change—rapid increase at the beginning and slower but continuing progress later—is similar for all strengthening exercises.

I found my clothing was getting bigger. I knew I needed something smaller, so I bought 14s. Then I had to take them back because I needed 12s and sometimes 10s. My arms got much firmer; my legs and hips got trimmer. People say I look great.

If you need to lose weight, strength training helps in three very important ways:

◆ GIVES YOUR METABOLISM A BOOST

Muscle is active tissue, so it consumes energy. Stored fat, on the other hand, is mostly inert; thus its energy requirements are very low. What does more muscle mean for dieters? More food! A higher calorie allowance makes it easier to stick to your eating plan—and you get more nutrients too.

Remember Bonnie, who was assigned to the nonexercise group in my *JAMA* study but began lifting weights afterward? Strength training helped her lose the fifteen pounds she gained when she quit smoking—and it's helped her maintain the loss, even under challenging circumstances:

> *I'm down from a size 12 to size 8, and I've kept it off even though I love to eat. When I took a five-day cruise, I went to the exercise room every day and used the equipment. Usually, if you go on a cruise and eat whatever you want, you gain weight. But I lost a pound.*

♦ Makes Aerobic Exercise More Enjoyable

As we all know, it's much easier to lose weight and keep it off if you're burning calories with exercise. Unfortunately, many overweight

Fast Twitch, Slow Twitch

You may have read about fast- and slow-twitch muscle fibers. The fibers that specialize in rapid movements and lifting heavy objects are called **fast-twitch.** Though they can move fast, they also become fatigued very quickly. Other fibers, **slow-twitch,** contract more slowly, but they're capable of working for a long time. The soleus muscles in the back of your calves, and other muscles used all day to maintain balance and posture, consist mainly of slow-twitch fibers.

One reason we become less capable of rapid movement as we get older is that the proportion of fast-twitch fibers in our bodies declines. Why this happens is a matter of controversy. Some investigators believe that we lose more fast-twitch than slow-twitch fibers with age. However, others speculate that these fibers aren't lost but are transformed into slow-twitch fibers as we become less active. This much is clear: Both aerobic exercise and strength training improve the performance of fast-twitch fibers, regardless of age.

women don't enjoy physical activity, even walking: It doesn't feel good; the extra weight is hard on their joints; and they're self-conscious about their bodies. Strength training is a great way to ease into aerobic exercise. We've found that when women start losing weight and become stronger, they often become more active in other ways—which further contributes to weight loss.

♦ ASSURES THAT YOU LOSE FAT, NOT MUSCLE

As I mentioned in Chapter 1, my colleagues and I did a small study in which we put overweight women on customized diets designed to let them lose weight gradually. One group simply followed the diet; the other also did strength training. Women in both groups lost about twenty pounds over the year of the study, as planned. However, the *composition* of the loss was different. Those in the diet-only group lost about five pounds of muscle. But the women who strength-trained maintained their muscle, so the pounds they dropped were truly excess fat. By the way, my second book, *Strong Women Stay Slim*, explains how to use the power of strength training for weight loss.

NOURISHING YOUR MUSCLES

You've probably seen the Food Pyramid, which summarizes the basic rules for healthy eating. If you follow these guidelines, your muscles will get all the nutrients they need—not only for strength training but for an active life. But many women fall short, even if they're nutrition-conscious. Review your food intake for the next three days. If you're like most of our volunteers, you'll probably discover plenty of room for improvement.

To maintain a healthy weight, select lower-fat meats, poultry, and dairy foods. Pay particular attention to serving sizes. Many are smaller than you might expect! Choose whole grains for the bread and cereal group to maximize satiety.

Here's how your muscles use the basic components of the food you eat:

◆ CARBOHYDRATE

Muscles draw quick energy from carbohydrates—glucose stored in the muscle and in the liver. This ready-to-use fuel supply is tapped when we need to move rapidly or to generate a lot of force. The "burn" you may feel in your muscles during strenuous exercise comes from the lactic acid that's produced when glucose is used.

◆ FAT

Fat is the other fuel source for muscle. It's less convenient than carbohydrate, because it must go through a series of metabolic processes to be used. On the other hand, our fat reserves are much larger, which means we can draw upon them for a sustained effort. The average woman has about 1,800 calories of stored carbohydrate, but her fat supply is 70,000 to 80,000

Food Guide Pyramid
A Guide to Daily Food Choices

Fats, Oils, & Sweets
USE SPARINGLY

KEY
☐ Fat (naturally occurring and added)   ▨ Sugars (added)
These symbols show that fat and added sugars come mostly from fats, oils, and sweets, but can be part of or added to foods from the other food groups as well.

Milk, Yogurt, & Cheese Group
2-3 SERVINGS

Meat, Poultry, Fish, Dry Beans, Eggs, & Nuts Group
2-3 SERVINGS

Vegetable Group
3-5 SERVINGS

Fruit Group
2-4 SERVINGS

Bread, Cereal, Rice, & Pasta Group
6-11 SERVINGS

SOURCE: U.S. Department of Agriculture/U.S. Department of Health and Human Services

WHAT COUNTS AS A SERVING
FOR THESE FOODS?

BREAD, CEREAL, RICE, AND PASTA
- 1 slice of bread
- 1 6-inch tortilla
- 1 cup of ready-to-eat cold cereal
- 1/2 cup of cooked cereal, rice, or pasta

VEGETABLES
- 1–2 cups of raw leafy vegetables
- 1/2 cup of other vegetables, cooked or chopped raw
- 3/4 cup of vegetable juice

FRUIT
- 1 medium apple, banana, or orange
- 1/2 cup of chopped, cooked, or canned fruit
- 3/4 cup of fruit juice

MILK, YOGURT, AND CHEESE
- 1 cup of milk or yogurt
- 1 ounce of natural cheese
- 2 ounces of processed cheese

MEAT, POULTRY, FISH, DRY BEANS, EGGS, AND NUTS
- 2–3 ounces of cooked lean meat, poultry, or fish
- 1/2 cup of cooked beans
- 1 egg, or 1 tablespoon of peanut butter = 1 ounce of meat

calories. Fat is our main fuel when we take an hour-long walk or play three sets of tennis.

◆ Protein

Myofibrils, the building blocks of muscle, are made up of protein. These cells constantly need repair or replacement. Indeed, our bodies renew about one pound of muscle tissue every day. Fortunately, about three-quarters of the necessary protein can be recycled in the renewal process, but we still need about a quarter of a pound of protein daily from our food. This can come from a variety of plant and animal sources.

You might assume that strength training, which builds muscle, would increase protein requirements, but careful laboratory measurements have shown it doesn't. Our newest studies have demonstrated that strength training actually enables the body to use protein more efficiently.

What about protein supplements? They're not necessary: No studies have demonstrated that they improve muscle size or strength. Indeed, excess protein can be harmful, because your kidneys have to work overtime to process the resulting wastes. What's more, there's evidence suggesting that excessive protein increases the loss of calcium from your bones.

NEW FINDINGS ABOUT MUSCLES AND HEALTH

I feel lucky to be working in such an exciting field. Every month, it seems, a new study uncovers yet another benefit of strength training. No surprise that gaining muscle makes you stronger and more energetic. And I've already explained how strength training can help you lose weight. But we're learning that the health implications are even broader. Here are three examples:

◆ Strength Training Helps Your Heart

Heart disease is the number-one killer of men and women. We all know that aerobic exercise is essential for cardiac health—and now we're

THE POWER CONNECTION

If you can lift a heavy weight, you're strong. But if you can lift it quickly, you've got power. Power combines strength and speed. Strong legs help you climb stairs—with powerful legs, you can take them two at a time. Until recently, we believed that power was important only for elite athletes, like sprinters or basketball players, whose activities require bursts of speed. But surprising new research suggests that power is vital for the elderly too.

My colleague Mona Foldvari, M.S., and her associates recently tested both power and strength in eighty frail older women. They compared the results with practical measures of independence, such as whether a woman needed assistance with everyday tasks like shopping, house cleaning, or bathing. The physical factor most closely related to independence was leg power. The next phase of the study involves exercise programs. We hope to learn if power training, or a combination of power and strength training, is more beneficial than strength training alone.

What about younger women—is power training important for them too? Most experts don't think so. We believe that active women under age seventy have all the power they need for daily life. Moreover, there's concern that power training—which often involves rapid weight lifting—could cause injuries, especially in women who aren't strong.

When a physically active woman tells me she wants to begin power training, I suggest lunges (see the supplemental exercises in Chapter 11) and short bursts of rapid stair climbing. These moves are safe for a woman who's already fit. If she's interested in going further, I urge her to work one-on-one with a certified personal trainer to make sure she learns appropriate moves and proper form. If a woman isn't active, I advise her to start strength-training and aerobic activity before power training.

discovering that strength training helps, too, because it makes your body leaner. And the better your muscle-to-fat ratio, the lower your risk of heart disease. Even individuals who already have cardiac problems can benefit from adding these exercises.

After our success with the frail elderly, Yael Beniamini, Ph.D., then a doctoral student in our laboratory, studied patients in a local cardiac rehabilitation program. Half got the usual care, including a walking program; the others also did strength training three times a week. After twelve weeks, the usual-care group was slightly stronger—but those who strength-trained showed dramatic increases. Moreover, their *aerobic* improvement was much greater, even though both groups had followed the same walking program.

◆ Strength Training Relieves Arthritis Symptoms

Who would have thought that people with arthritis could lift weights? It turns out they can—and what's more, strength training actually brings relief! Ronenn Roubenoff, M.D., M.H.S., chief of our laboratory, demonstrated benefits for individuals with moderate to severe rheumatoid arthritis. Though walking and other weight-bearing exercise was painful for these volunteers, they were able to strength-train. The findings were very encouraging: Strength training decreased their pain and improved their range of motion. The program also restored strength and muscle, which is especially important for people with arthritis—often they lose muscle because pain keeps them inactive or because they're taking muscle-depleting drugs, such as corticosteroids.

Kristin Baker, Ph.D., other colleagues, and I found similar gains in men and women with osteoarthritis of the knee. After four months of at-home exercises similar to those in this book, the volunteers reported an average 43 percent reduction in pain. They scored 40 percent higher on our tests of joint function and a whopping 50 percent higher on strength. Also encouraging were their improvements in self-confidence and overall well-being.

◆ ◆ ◆

I suffered a stroke at age fifty-two in 1993. Thanks to your book, I am now physically stronger—and for the first time

since my stroke, I am emotionally strong. The exercises helped almost immediately, but when I reached twelve pounds, there was a miraculous improvement. I can do without my ankle brace. I am able to clean house without crying in pain. I substitute teach, and it is much easier now to get through a school day.
   —Miriam

Having high blood pressure, fibromyalgia, and arthritis in my left knee, I had been feeling old—at forty-three. The future didn't look very bright. I wanted you to know that I have been progressing with the Strong Women *program. I find it easier to get out of bed each morning and keep moving. Although I still have days when all my muscles ache, for the first time in about six years I feel that the fibromyalgia is in retreat.*
   —Monica

Eight years ago after the birth of my first baby (age thirty), I was told by my neurologist that I had MS. I had great difficulty lifting, walking, and the like. Your book sounded like everything I needed. After three or four weeks I was carrying in the groceries with my daughters' help. Previously I could lift no more than one jug. This time, when I walked into the kitchen, my oldest daughter said, "Mom, look at you!" I had two jugs in one hand and a ten-pound bag of potatoes in the other! In the spring we went to Zion National Park. Not only did I hike one of the two-mile trails, but I ran! I even carried my six-year-old daughter part of the way. My MS symptoms have not gone away, but strength training has helped me keep them under control. I feel great!
   —Jean

♦ ♦ ♦

♦ STRENGTH TRAINING LIFTS DEPRESSION

You probably know that aerobic exercise is a wonderfully healthy way to boost your spirits. We've found that strength training has the same effect. Some of Dr. Maria Fiatarone's nursing home volunteers suffered from depression when they entered her program. As the weeks passed and they grew stronger, she noticed that they seemed much happier. So she and a colleague, Nalin Singh, M.D., conducted a separate investigation to see if strength training could improve mood.

Thirty-two men and women, who met clinical guidelines for depression, were assigned at random to a strength-training program or to a discussion group. Ten weeks later, people receiving both treatments showed improvement—not surprising, since everyone got supportive attention. However, the change was significantly greater for the sixteen participants who exercised. Fourteen of them—but just eight of those in the discussion group—no longer met the criteria for clinical depression. This dramatic difference is comparable to results from highly effective antidepressant medications, but without all the side effects. We don't yet know if strength training helps because people feel good about being stronger, or if the explanation involves helpful biochemical changes in the brains. Most likely, it's a combination.

♦ ♦ ♦

Strength training makes me feel very physical and very competent. It makes me feel I'm strong and coordinated. I never thought of myself that way, because I was always chosen last for sports—and it's great.
—Lisa

♦ ♦ ♦

To Read More About Nutrition

Strong Women Stay Slim (Bantam, 1998) includes two chapters on nutrition, with scientific research and practical advice about weight loss; a flexible food plan that follows the Food Guide Pyramid; plus menus and recipes by renowned food writer Steven Raichlen.

For up-to-date information, I recommend the monthly *Tufts University Health & Nutrition Letter* (P.O. Box 420235, Palm Coast, FL 32142-0235; telephone 1-800-274-7581 or 1-904-447-2837).

Here are five excellent books that provide practical, accurate information on nutrition:

- *The Tufts University Guide to Total Nutrition* (updated), by Stanley Gershoff, Ph.D., with Catherine Whitney (Harper Perennial, 1996).
- *The American Dietetic Association Guide to Women's Nutrition for Healthy Living*, by Susan Calvert Finn and Janet Grant Tougas (Perigee, 1997).
- *The Wellness Encyclopedia of Food and Nutrition*, by Sheldon Margen, M.D., and the editors of the *University of California at Berkeley Wellness Letter* (Rebus, 1992).
- *Jane Brody's Good Food Book*, by Jane Brody (Bantam, 1985).
- *Nancy Clark's Sports Nutrition Guidebook*, by Nancy Clark, M.S., R.D. (Human Kinetics, 1996).

Here are three recommended online sources of nutrition information:

- The Tufts University Nutrition Navigator (http://navigator.tufts.edu) has links to hundreds of nutrition and health resources.
- American Dietetic Association (http://www.eatright.org) provides nutrition fact sheets (many with delicious recipes) and can put you in touch with ADA's "Find a dietitian" service. Or call 1-800-336-1655.
- Cyberdiet (http://www.cyberdiet.com) offers nutrition information, recipes, assessment tools, and a variety of support groups.

BONING UP ON
YOUR SKELETON

◆ ◆ ◆

I visited my sister, who's fifteen years older and lives in California. She has osteoporosis. I was in total shock to see that she was about half my height. All of a sudden I was worried about my bones. I knew I needed to do something.
    —Verna

I'm still a few years away from menopause, but hormone replacement therapy is already on my mind and it makes my head spin. Sure, I'd love to stick a patch on my rear end that would ward off osteoporosis and heart disease. But my mother, her sister, and most of their cousins had breast cancer, and frankly, that scares me even more. It's such a relief to know I can help my bones without fear of harming my breasts!
    —Jayne

◆ ◆ ◆

became interested in bones when I was growing up because every spring, for four years in a row, I broke a bone. When I was eight years old, I fell off a pony and broke my shoulder. The next year I smashed my ankle in a car accident. The following spring I crushed part of my spine in gymnastics, and a year later, also in gymnastics, I broke a bone in my foot. While I was recovering I asked the doctors a lot of questions, and I remember vividly how their answers fascinated me. This is one reason I eventually wound up doing bone research.

Because I was a child when I had this series of injuries, my bones healed quickly. But I certainly don't take bone health for granted. Three of my favorite relatives have osteoporosis: Two of my in-laws have broken their hips, and my aunt suffers from constant pain because of osteoporotic fractures in her spine. Because of my family history, I'm tremendously encouraged by recent advances in this area. My research and other studies have shown how much we can do to keep our bones strong. And women have new options for treating bone loss that weren't available just a few years ago.

A CLOSER LOOK AT BONE

Your body contains over two hundred bones, joined by cartilage and ligaments. Together they form your skeleton, the framework that supports and protects your muscles and internal organs.

When you touch your bones through soft skin, they feel as solid and unchanging as rock. But that's just the outer shell. Underneath, bone tissue is porous and very much alive. Blood vessels run through it and at the center is bone marrow, where blood cells are formed.

Bone is made of calcium and other minerals—that's why it's hard. Like muscle, bone tissue constantly repairs and renews itself, though with bone this happens much more slowly. The process, called **remodeling,** is the work of two kinds of cells:

- **Osteoclasts** break down damaged bone, releasing calcium into the blood.
- **Osteoblasts** draw calcium from the blood and create new bone.

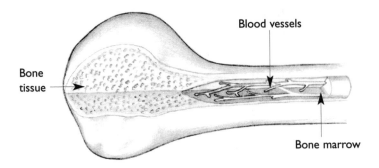

Blood vessels

Bone tissue

Bone marrow

Remodeling is affected by many factors, but the three most important are:

♦ ESTROGEN AND OTHER HORMONES

Estrogen restrains the bone-dissolving activity of the osteoclasts. The brakes let up after menopause, when the ovaries produce less estrogen. The osteoblasts keep building, but their efforts are outdone by the out-of-control osteoclasts. So there's a net loss of bone.

♦ CALCIUM SUPPLY AND DEMAND

Calcium is essential to many of the body's behind-the-scenes chemical reactions—it's needed for muscles to contract, to regulate blood pressure, and to control bleeding. If you don't get enough calcium from your diet, your body is forced to draw on the supply stored in your bones.

♦ MECHANICAL FORCES

Physical impact stimulates bone formation. That's why walking is a better exercise for bones than swimming: When you float in water, you barely touch bottom, but when you walk, your feet hit against the ground. The tug of muscle against bone works the same way. This is one reason that strength training affects bone density. And the stronger your muscles, the more stimulation they provide.

THE LIFE CYCLE AND YOUR BONES

Your bones grow through your entire life. But over the years, the balance shifts between building and breaking down.

From birth to twenty-five
Remodeling works in your favor, and you add more bone than you lose. Bone mass is at its maximum around age twenty-five.

Age twenty-five to thirty-five
If you're healthy, you maintain bone density, neither gaining nor losing.

Age thirty-five to menopause
You reach a turning point. For the first time in your life, your natural tendency is to lose bone—up to 1 percent each year. If you don't take measures to prevent it, you'll undergo the transformation called **osteopenia,** from *osteo* for "bone" and *penia* meaning "loss." It's similar to sarcopenia (muscle loss), which I discussed in Chapter 2.

The first five years after menopause
During this short period—unless you do something about it—you'll lose 1 to 2 percent or even more of your bone mass every year. **This is the most critical time for preventive measures.**

Age fifty-five to seventy
Bone loss slows down—thank goodness! But you still lose an average of about 1 percent per year.

Age seventy and older
The average rate of loss slows further, to less than half a percent a year.

Can Osteoporosis Affect Teeth?

Yes! Doctors and dentists have assumed that older people lose teeth because of gum disease. They're just beginning to realize that the culprit is often bone loss. It makes sense: When bone in the jaw becomes less dense, teeth aren't held as securely. So they may loosen and even fall out.

OSTEOPOROSIS: SILENT SABOTAGE

If bone loss isn't interrupted—and it can be—the result is osteoporosis, a condition in which bones become dangerously fragile. Osteoporosis affects about 28 million Americans, mostly women, and many of them don't know it. How can a woman tell if she's crossed the line? Most often she finds out when she falls, and instead of winding up with a bruise, she breaks a bone. Or her doctor makes the diagnosis when she scores significantly below normal on a bone density test.

Another sign is diminished height. Have you ever wondered why so many people get shorter and bent over as they get older? It's *not* bad posture. This happens because fragile, osteoporotic vertebrae, bones in their spine, get crushed. Women may not realize what's happening because these fractures don't always hurt right away. My aunt, who's now in her seventies, probably started losing bone in her late thirties. Only decades later did the treacherous disease become evident. Today this formerly energetic, fun-loving woman has lost her zest. She spends most of the day lying down or sitting, trying to get comfortable.

For a young woman, a broken bone is painful and inconvenient but it heals fast. The consequences are far more serious for someone older. Each year about 300,000 people wind up in hospitals with hip fractures because of osteoporosis. This is a devastating injury: Half of its victims never go home again, and one in five dies from complications within a year. Even if a woman is lucky enough to survive, even if she doesn't wind up in a nursing home, she may lose her independence because she's so fearful of falling again.

The Fracture Zone

If bone loss isn't stopped, a woman enters the **fracture zone:** Her bones become so fragile that they could break not only if she falls, but even from ordinary activities. "I bent down to put food in a bowl for my cat, something I've done every day for the past seventeen years," an eighty-six-year-old woman told me. "And I crushed a vertebra in my spine."

If you look at the photos on page 48, which show magnified pictures of healthy bone and of osteoporotic bone in the fracture zone, it's easy to see how that could happen. What a difference! The normal bone is porous and looks like the sturdy lattice of a bridge. But the osteoporotic bone is more air than substance.

I want to emphasize that there's more to the fracture zone than bone density, important as that is. Most osteoporotic fractures are caused by falls, and elderly women fall because they lose their balance easily and aren't strong enough to recover. For them, even ordinary moves can lead to falls—turning too quickly, reaching on tiptoe for something on a high shelf. Muscles and balance can protect whatever bone a woman has. That's why strengthening exercises are so critical.

Are You at Risk?

The likelihood that you'll get osteoporosis depends on many factors, some preventable and some not. These are the unavoidable risk factors:

- ◆ **Gender:** The risk is much greater because you're a woman.
- ◆ **Age:** The older you are, the greater the risk.

Healthy bone is not a matter of age.

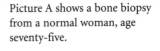

Picture A shows a bone biopsy from a normal woman, age seventy-five.

Picture B is the bone of a much younger woman, age forty-seven, who has osteoporosis.

- **Race:** The lighter your skin, the greater the risk. Caucasian and Asian women have a higher incidence of osteoporotic fractures than African-American and Hispanic women.
- **Family history:** If your mother or grandmother had low bone density and osteoporotic fractures, you're at higher risk.
- **Body type:** The smaller your frame, the greater your risk. Thinner women have a higher risk than heavier women.
- **Early menopause:** If you reached menopause before age forty-five—whether naturally or because your ovaries were removed—you're at greater risk.

Are you vulnerable? If so, it's especially important to pay attention to the risk factors you *can* avoid:

- **Sedentary lifestyle:** The less active you are, the higher your risk. Conversely, increasing activity lowers the danger. This is in part because exercise builds stronger bones and muscles, and improves balance.
- **Menstrual interruptions:** If you've had menstrual interruptions (other than pregnancy) before menopause, you're at elevated risk. The most common causes are eating disorders (anorexia or bulimia) or excessive exercise combined with an inadequate diet. Ironically, this category includes apparently vigorous women athletes and dancers.
- **Poor diet:** Your bones suffer if you don't eat well. Calcium and vitamin D are especially important.
- **Cigarette smoking:** Yet another reason to quit: Women who smoke have lower bone density and also lose bone more rapidly after age forty.
- **Drinking:** A little alcohol is fine, but a lot—more than seven drinks per week—interferes with calcium metabolism and thereby hurts your bones.

The more the odds are stacked against you by both unavoidable and avoidable risk factors, the more important prevention—including strength training—becomes.

Medical Treatments That Can Hurt Your Bones

Illness and medical treatment can affect bones. Doctors correctly focus their attention on the main problem, so they may need a reminder that bone health is important too.

CANCER TREATMENT

Chemotherapy can be difficult and debilitating. Your bones may suffer not only from the drugs but also from inactivity and inability to eat well. When you're finished with treatment and feel up to starting an exercise program, talk to your doctor about how you can recover the muscle and bone you lost during chemotherapy.

LONG-TERM USE OF CERTAIN MEDICATIONS

If you're taking drugs for a chronic medical condition, your bones could be affected. Read the package insert, and talk to your doctor if there's a potential problem—you may be able to lower the dose or switch to a different drug. The medications below can weaken bones:

- Steroids (prednisone, for example), used for asthma and arthritis
- Thyroid hormones
- Barbiturates and anticonvulsants, used to prevent seizures or to treat certain cardiac irregularities
- Antacids containing aluminum
- Methotrexate, used for arthritis, cancer, psoriasis, and immune disorders

CHECK OUT YOUR BONES

At this point, you're probably wondering how healthy your bones are. You could take a test to find out, but it's expensive and not all women need it. However, bone density testing is something to consider under the following circumstances:

◆ You have a risk factor for osteoporosis other than age, sex, and race. Jill—who's five feet ten inches tall and weighs about 135 pounds—plans to be tested:

I'm forty-eight now and really worry about osteoporosis. My mother has it and so did her older sister, who was my favorite aunt. She fractured her hip last spring, developed complications, and died seven weeks later. After the funeral we were looking at family pictures. At my college graduation party she was tall, only an inch shorter than me. But the last time I saw her, a few weeks before she died, she didn't even reach my chin.

◆ You're about to undergo a medical treatment (including treatment for osteoporosis) that might affect your bones. This would enable your doctor to monitor changes. For example, I'd suggest a baseline test for a woman who's about to have her ovaries removed or who's just started long-term steroid treatment for arthritis.

◆ You're trying to decide about hormone replacement therapy. Jill's grandmother had breast cancer, so she'd rather not take estrogen. Should she do it for her bones? A test will help her weigh the risks and benefits with her doctor.

Several techniques are used to measure bone density:

◆ **Dual energy X-ray absorptiometry** (DXA or DEXA) is the best test and is widely available—we used it in my *JAMA* study. It's painless and quick and can measure density of the spine and hip bones as well as total body bone density. Another important advantage is very low radiation exposure—so little, in fact, that the technician can remain right next to the scanner during the test instead of leaving the room. The cost is $200 to $300; insurance may cover it. Since DXA scanners are calibrated differently, it's best to return to the same place for any subsequent tests or the results may not be comparable.

♦ **Ultrasound** tests are now commonly available. They're quick and inexpensive ($30 to $100) and involve no radiation. Ultrasound can measure bone density in the heel and hand, which is a good indicator of overall bone health. But it's not a substitute for direct measurement of spine and hip bone density by DXA.

♦ **Single energy X-ray absorptiometry** measures bone density at the heel or wrist but not at the hip and spine, which are more important. However, it may be less expensive than DXA, and the measurements of the heel and wrist are a useful indicator of overall bone health.

♦ **Quantitative computed tomography** (CT scan) can measure the hip and spine, but this test is more expensive than DXA and entails more radiation exposure.

♦ **X-rays** can spot a fracture but can't measure bone density as precisely as the other tests.

WHY DON'T MEN HAVE THIS PROBLEM?

Men don't really escape the fracture zone, as I'll explain in Chapter 13. They just take a lot longer to get there. I can name more than a dozen older women friends and relatives who have broken their bones, but only a few men. If you think about the people you know, the numbers probably are similar. Here's why:

Men don't live as long as we do, but nature has blessed them with more bone mineral and stronger muscles. They enter the second half of life with ample bone reserves thanks in part to testosterone (the male hormone), which stimulates bone and muscle growth, and in part to diet—they eat more than we do and therefore get more calcium. Men also tend to be more active, which builds up bone and muscle too. Another difference: Testosterone levels decline with age, but men experience nothing like the drop in estrogen we have with menopause. So even though men lose bone too, it usually doesn't become a problem until they reach their eighties.

Women, in contrast, are hit with a triple whammy: We start out with less bone; at around age fifty we lose a lot in a short time; and we're not as muscular. So we're much more likely to reach the danger point at an earlier age.

PREVENTING OSTEOPOROSIS

Building bone mass is like putting money in the bank: The sooner you start, the more you'll have later in life. But no matter what your age, there's a lot you can do now to protect your bones. The greater your risk, the more important these preventive measures:

- ◆ Make sure you get enough calcium and vitamin D; take supplements if necessary.
- ◆ Do strengthening exercise to build bone and to reduce the risk of falls. If you're at high risk or actually have osteoporosis, consider joining a gym so you can strength-train on machines. Because your body is held in the correct position by the machine, you can safely lift heavier weights that way. (See Chapter 12 for a gym-based strength-training program.)
- ◆ Get plenty of weight-bearing aerobic exercise—walking is ideal—because that helps protect bone.
- ◆ Consider balance training to reduce the chance of falls.
- ◆ Discuss bone density testing with your doctor, especially if you know you're at risk.
- ◆ If you're at high risk or already have osteoporosis, talk to your doctor about medication, which can be extraordinarily helpful.

THE POWER OF STRENGTH

I've already mentioned that astronauts became weak in the early days of the space program. They also lost bone. This raised an interesting question: If bones suffered from idleness in a weightless environment, might they benefit from hard work? To find out, investigators looked at people who challenged their bones.

One study compared the left and right arm bones of professional tennis players. It turned out that bones in their racket arms were 15 to 20 percent denser than bones in their other arms. Another study found unusually thick hand bones in lumberjacks who used chain saws. Of course, these associations didn't prove that activity *caused* bone growth. After all, it could be that people with thick hand bones are especially likely to pick lumberjacking as a career. So scientists recruited volunteers, put them on carefully controlled exercise programs, and measured the effects.

My *JAMA* study was part of this effort. I knew from other research that a strong relationship exists between the amount of muscle in a person's body and the amount of bone. My hypothesis, which the study confirmed, was that increasing muscle mass would increase bone density as well. The women in our study were all postmenopausal; none was taking estrogen or other bone-strengthening medication, or consuming an unusually high amount of calcium. Nevertheless, those in the strength-training group *gained* an average of 1 percent of bone density in the hip and spine—comparable to the bone benefit from hormone replacement therapy. Women in the control group *lost* 2 to 2.5 percent.

We knew that strength training would make women stronger, and the study confirmed that as well. But we were surprised at how much our volunteers' balance improved, and we did not expect their activity level to leap by 27 percent. These results are very exciting because they mean that **one simple intervention can not only reverse bone loss but also decrease other risk factors for osteoporotic fractures.**

CALCIUM—AND VITAMIN D— FOR STRONG BONES

All the calcium in our bones comes from the food we eat. So if we don't get enough, we endanger our bones. But calcium alone is not sufficient. Without vitamin D, our bodies can't use the calcium we consume. Below are the latest recommendations for daily calcium and vitamin D—now called the Dietary Reference Intake (DRI)—from the Institute of Medicine at the National Academy of Sciences. And you'll find a list of calcium-rich foods on the next two pages.

DIETARY REFERENCE INTAKE		
FOR WOMEN AND MEN	CALCIUM (MG/DAY)	VITAMIN D (IU/DAY)
Age		
Birth to 6 months	210	200
6 months to 1 year	270	200
1 to 3	500	200
4 to 8	800	200
9 to 18	1300	200
19 to 50	1000	200
51 to 70	1200	400
71 and older	1200	600
If pregnant or lactating		
Under age 19	1300	200
19 and older	1000	200

Calcium-Rich Foods

Food	Portion	Calcium (mg)
Dairy products		
Milk (whole, 2%, 1%, or skim)	8 ounces	300
Ricotta cheese, part skim	4 ounces	250-350
Cheddar cheese	1 ounce	200
Cottage cheese	4 ounces	60-80
Yogurt (plain or flavored)	8 ounces	275-325
Ice cream, frozen yogurt	4 ounces	70-120
Milk-based puddings and custards	4 ounces	150
Nondairy products		
Calcium-fortified orange juice	8 ounces	200-300
Bean curd (tofu) with calcium sulfate	1/2 cup	250

FOOD	PORTION	CALCIUM (MG)
Nondairy products (*cont.*)		
Soy milk (calcium-fortified)	8 ounces	200–300
Spinach, cooked	1/2 cup	125
Other leafy greens (mustard greens, kale, bok choy, cabbage), cooked	1/2 cup	50
Leafy greens, raw	1 cup	50
Other vegetables (broccoli, green beans, squash), cooked	1/2 cup	30
Beans, cooked	1 cup	50-120
Salmon (canned, with bones)	3 ounces	200
Rhubarb, cooked	1/2 cup	175

Calcium

The best dietary sources of calcium are dairy foods. But there are alternatives.

When I show the chart on pages 56 and 57 at lectures, the hands fly up. These are the questions I get most frequently:

"What if I don't like milk?"

Dairy products aren't the only dietary source of calcium, but they're by far the richest. You can get about half of the calcium you need by drinking just two glasses of milk a day. When a woman tells me she doesn't like milk, I sympathize, because I feel the same way. Yet if we start talking, and I ask what she likes to eat, often it turns out that she's happy to have breakfast cereal with milk; she enjoys creamy soups and casseroles; she snacks on cheddar cheese—and her favorite desserts are yogurt and ice cream. I get most of my calcium from dairy foods like these, as well as from broccoli and other vegetables. And just to make sure I'm getting enough, I drink calcium-fortified orange juice.

"How do I get enough calcium if I don't eat any foods that come from animals?"

No doubt about it, women who abstain from all dairy products have more difficulty getting the calcium they need from food. But it is possible. Tofu that's made with calcium sulfate is a great source—check the label. Other good sources are listed on pages 56 and 57.

"I like dairy products, but my body can't tolerate them— what should I do?"

A small number of people are allergic to the protein in milk. If you have this problem, you may be able to eat cheese or dairy foods that have been cooked, since heat denatures the protein.

A more common difficulty is lactose intolerance. If you lack the enzyme needed to digest lactose, the natural sugar in milk, dairy products may give you gas, cramps, or diarrhea. These suggestions might help:

- Try reducing portions of dairy foods—many people who consider themselves lactose intolerant can, in fact, drink milk in smaller amounts, such as half a cup several times a day.
- Add the enzyme (called lactase) to milk or other dairy foods, or buy milk to which it is already added. Health food stores—and, increasingly, regular supermarkets—sell these products, usually in the dairy case.
- Eat yogurt made with live cultures (check the label)—they break down the lactose for you.
- Get calcium from cheese; the manufacturing process breaks down lactose.

Vitamin D

Vitamin D comes from two sources: diet and the sun, which triggers cells in the skin to manufacture the vitamin.

The best food sources are fortified milk and fortified cereal. But most women don't get enough vitamin D from food. If you're outside daily during summer months, you'll meet your vitamin D requirement in just ten minutes. But it's difficult—and even impossible for those who live in a northern state or province—to get enough exposure in the winter. That's because the angle of the sun's rays changes and can't trigger the necessary reaction in the skin. For instance, because I live in Boston, I can't get my vitamin D from the sun from November to February. Because of this, women in these climates lose 2 to 4 percent of their bone in the winter; if they're young and healthy, they gain all of it back in the summer.

What About Supplements?

Experts agree that it's better to get nutrients from food if possible. No vitamin or mineral pill can replace a well-rounded diet for the following reasons:

◆ Scientists haven't yet pinpointed all the beneficial nutrients that foods contain. So if we rely on supplements, we may miss out. One example is lycopene, which is a phytochemical—a compound found naturally in plants. This nutrient made headlines when Harvard researchers discovered a lower-than-average incidence of prostate cancer in men who eat tomatoes. The benefit seems to come from lycopene, which is present in tomatoes but not (so far) in vitamin pills.

◆ It's nearly impossible to get too much calcium and vitamin D from food—but this can happen with supplements. Excessive calcium may interfere with absorption of iron and zinc, two other very important minerals.

◆ Nutrients in food generally are more bioavailable. For example, if we get small amounts of calcium all through the day in meals and snacks, rather than a single large dose in pill form, it's easier for our bodies to use it. Also, calcium is more readily absorbed when it's dissolved and accompanied by natural sugars.

◆　◆　◆

I talked to my doctor about osteoporosis at my last checkup. She questioned me about my diet and told me I should be getting more calcium. I'd been reading about supplements and knew bioavailability was an issue. So I asked if there was a brand of calcium supplements available in liquid form with natural sugars. She said, "Yes. It's called 'milk.'"
—*Jill*

◆　◆　◆

If you can't get all the calcium and vitamin D that you need from food, I suggest you take a supplement to help protect your bones. Here are some recommendations:

- Select a brand that contains both calcium and 400 IU of vitamin D.
- Both calcium carbonate and calcium citrate are good supplements, but calcium citrate has a slight edge because it's easier to absorb.
- Choose an appropriate dose. Take into account the calcium and vitamin D you consume in your diet. There's no need to go above the optimum (see page 55). Indeed, you might have digestive problems if you do.
- Take the supplement in the evening—after dinner or before bedtime. Your digestive system moves more slowly at night, which will allow the calcium and vitamin D more time to be absorbed.

ESTROGEN

◆ ◆ ◆

My mother has osteoporosis. Now that I'm entering menopause, she's after me to start hormones. But I don't want to take a drug every day for the rest of my life if I don't have to. I heard your interview on the public radio station, so I'm writing to ask if there's anything else I can do instead.
—Fax from a forty-nine-year-old woman in Australia

I have to decide about estrogen. Half my friends are taking it; the other half say "No way!" Every week I read something different. My doctor is gung-ho; he thinks it's the greatest thing since penicillin. I keep going back and forth. What do you think?
—Comment from a fifty-three-year-old woman at a lecture

◆ ◆ ◆

These questions are typical of the hundreds I get each year in letters, phone calls, and at lectures. Women are being buffeted by all the claims and counterclaims about estrogen. They worry about taking hormones, and they worry about *not* taking them and possibly shortchanging themselves later in life. This question concerns nearly all of us. I don't have any simple answers, but I can offer information and two general recommendations:

- ◆ First: Hormone replacement therapy (HRT) involves both benefits and risks, and these are not the same for all individuals. This is a personal decision that you should make with a very well-informed physician who knows your medical history. What's right for your best friend isn't necessarily what's right for you.
- ◆ Second: Whether or not you take estrogen, strength training and aerobic exercise will help protect your bones and your heart—and they're virtually risk free.

HRT offers very important benefits. It significantly reduces a woman's risk of osteoporosis and bone fractures; it also offers protection against heart disease and probably against Alzheimer's disease too. Taking estrogen (usually in combination with progesterone) for a few months or a year or two during the change of life can ease normal menopausal symptoms such as hot flashes, mood swings, vaginal dryness, and sleep disruptions.

All these benefits last as long as the woman continues HRT. But there are trade-offs. Many women experience side effects, including breakthrough bleeding or spotting, water retention, breast tenderness, and cramps. Also, long-term use of HRT increases the risk of breast cancer. The dilemma was underscored by a major report in 1995, based on data from a Harvard study that has been monitoring the health of over 100,000 nurses since the mid-1970s. About 70,000 of the nurses are now post-menopausal. Those who have taken HRT for ten years or more have half the usual rate of heart attacks and hip fractures—very impressive benefits to their hearts and bones. But the price is a significantly higher rate of breast cancer starting after five years of HRT.

Because of the benefits, I believe that HRT should be considered by most post-menopausal women who are not at elevated risk for breast cancer. The decision is easier for women whose medical histories point in a single direction. HRT is nearly always recommended for women who have menopause before age forty-five or whose ovaries are surgically removed; otherwise there's a real risk that their skeletons won't last as long as the rest of their bodies. If a woman has a strong family history of both heart disease and osteoporosis, her doctor probably will recommend HRT. On the other hand, if her mother died of breast cancer at age fifty-five, the doctor might advise against it.

Even if you take HRT, you still can benefit from strength training. Morris Notelovitz, M.D., Ph.D., from the Women's Medical and Diagnostic Center in Gainesville, Florida, studied women who had been on HRT for at least six months after their ovaries were removed. All continued taking estrogen, but half also did strength training for a year. At the end of the study, the HRT-only group had maintained their bone density. But the women who had strength-trained *gained* bone—an average of 4 percent in their wrists and 8 percent in their spines. Because they also became stronger and improved their balance—and therefore were less likely to fall—their risk of osteoporotic fractures was dramatically lower than if they'd relied on estrogen alone.

TREATING OSTEOPOROSIS

Women with osteoporosis now have promising treatment options that didn't exist before the mid-1990s. And the list grows steadily.

Until 1985 hormone replacement was the only treatment for osteoporosis. Calcitonin came along in 1985. Though this medication also preserved bone, the side effects, including nausea and flushing of the face or hands, were a problem for many women.

In 1995, a new drug, called alendronate (brand name Fosamax), received approval from the Food and Drug Administration. Alendronate is a nonhormonal medicine that suppresses the activity of osteoclasts, the cells that break down bone. Numerous clinical trials have shown that it can increase bone density substantially, reducing spine and hip fractures by about 50 percent in women with osteoporosis. Though it too can have side effects, including nausea and indigestion, most women can tolerate the drug if they take it with plenty of fluid on an empty stomach.

CAN TESTOSTERONE PROTECT WOMEN'S BONES?

Testosterone is the male hormone, but women have small amounts of it too. Since men's higher testosterone levels help protect them from osteoporosis, you may wonder—as have doctors and scientists—if a little extra would benefit women as well. The bottom line: We don't yet know.

Though the Food and Drug Administration has approved testosterone for treatment of menopausal symptoms, it is *not* yet approved for osteoporosis. Preliminary evidence suggests that testosterone, combined with estrogen, is slightly more effective than estrogen alone in improving bone density. Estrogen protects bone by blocking the action of osteoclasts, the cells that break down bone. Adding testosterone seems to increase bone formation.

Offsetting this potential benefit are troubling side effects. These can include: weight gain, voice lowering, acne, facial hair, and increased body odor.

At the moment, there's not enough evidence for me to recommend that you take testosterone to protect your bones. But research is ongoing—and worth watching.

In the mid-1990s, breast cancer researchers noticed that women taking tamoxifen were experiencing an unexpected positive side effect: bone preservation. Tamoxifen is a selective estrogen receptor modulator (SERM), a drug that doesn't actually add estrogen but makes the body more receptive to existing supplies. This type of drug is sometimes called a "weak estrogen" because it has mild estrogenlike effects. SERMs apparently stimulate bone formation, but because they're less potent, they're much less likely to cause the troubling side effects that can occur with estrogen. The tamoxifen findings encouraged research on the bone-protective potential of other SERMs.

In 1998 the FDA approved raloxifen (Evista) for preventing osteoporosis, the first SERM to be used for this purpose. In 1999 raloxifen was approved for treatment as well. Meanwhile, other promising drugs are under investigation and should earn FDA approval within a few years.

I recommend strengthening exercises, along with medication, to women with osteoporosis. While we don't yet know if strength training boosts the bone benefits of newer drugs, as Dr. Notelovitz's research proved for HRT, I suspect we'll find that it does. In addition, strength training does something no osteoporosis medication can: It reduces the risk of falling by improving balance and strength.

My mother-in-law is a wonderful example. She broke her hip at age seventy-one and began strengthening exercises as part of her recovery. That was nine years ago. She's now eighty and stronger than she was before the fracture, with a lifestyle that would exhaust many women half her age. She helps run a vegetable farm in New Hampshire; she cross-country-skis with her grandchildren in the winter, and she swims and hikes with them in the summer. After the blizzards of 1996, she climbed onto the roof of her house to shovel off the snow. This is definitely *not* an activity I would recommend for a woman in her late seventies who's had a hip fracture! But her vitality is an inspiration—and a testimony to both her positive outlook and her strengthening exercises.

For More Information About Osteoporosis

My new book, *Strong Women, Strong Bones*, contains the latest scientific information about osteoporosis, plus practical advice on nutrition, exercise, and medication. To get additional help and updates, contact the following organizations:

National Osteoporosis Foundation
1232 22nd Street, N.W.
Washington, DC 20037-1292
Tel: 1-800-223-9994 or 1-202-223-2226
http://www.nof.org

Osteoporosis and Related Bone Diseases Resource Center
National Institutes of Health
1232 22nd Street, N.W.
Washington, DC 20037-1292
Tel: 1-800-624-BONE (2663) or 1-202-223-0344
http://www.osteo.org

Foundation for Osteoporosis Research and Education (FORE)
300 27th Street, Suite 103
Oakland, CA 94612
Tel: 1-888-266-3015 or 1-510-832-2663
http://www.fore.org

4

KEEPING
YOUR BALANCE

◆ ◆ ◆

I had excellent balance as a child. I could ride a bike when I was five; I could walk on stilts. I'm not aware of having poorer balance now, but something must be happening at the subconscious level because without thinking about it, I'm becoming more careful. If I go down stairs, I hold the railing. If I use a step stool, I position it next to something I can hang on to.
—Jayne

Before I started strength training, I used to fall onto my bed when I tried to get into the second leg of my pantyhose. Flopping over in that helpless fashion really bugged me. Well, now I can stand on one leg and maneuver quite comfortably.
—Ursula

◆ ◆ ◆

BALANCE TEST

Try this test: Close your eyes, and—for safety—hold your hands just above a firm support, such as a sturdy chair or countertop. Then, keeping your eyes shut, slowly lift one foot and try to balance on the other leg. Count the seconds you remain balanced.

If you're like most women past age forty, you'll be astonished to discover that you can't hold the position for even fifteen seconds.

Once we're past the childhood milestones of learning to walk and ride a bicycle, most of us take our balance for granted. Yet we rely upon this ability constantly—walking on an uneven lawn, pivoting if our name is called, reaching over a supermarket shopping cart to grab a cereal box.

We now know that balance starts to decline when we're in our forties. This happens so slowly that it's almost imperceptible. But if nothing is done to counter the changes, we'll become very much aware of diminished balance in our seventies and eighties.

Picture an elderly woman walking down the street, her gait slow and hesitant. Now imagine the confident stride of a young adult. Balance is what makes the difference. Older people unconsciously change how they walk to compensate for poor balance: They take shorter steps to avoid standing on just one foot; they shuffle to keep their feet close to the ground; they place their feet wider apart to give themselves a larger base of support.

Despite their precautions, about 30 percent of people over age sixty-five report at least one fall each year. Ten to 15 percent of these falls cause serious injuries. As you know from the previous chapter, an accident that might merely bruise a woman with strong bones can have devastating consequences for someone with osteoporosis. Poor balance affects even those who never actually get hurt. Because the risk is so fearsome, many older men and women curtail their physical activities just to avoid falling.

One of my most exciting findings is that strengthening exercise can improve balance. This combination of benefits—lowered risk of falling, combined with improved strength and bone density—makes strength training a highly promising way to ward off osteoporotic fractures.

HOW WE KEEP IN BALANCE

I'm fascinated by the exquisitely engineered system that enables us to remain upright whether we're moving or standing still. I appreciate my balance not only when I'm headed down a ski slope but in everyday life. Sometimes when I'm standing in a slow line at a store, I pay attention to the complex, subtle adjustments that happen automatically: I lean forward a fraction of an inch, and my body corrects by leaning back; someone accidentally bumps me with a shopping bag, and I teeter slightly but quickly right myself again.

The parts of the brain that govern movement also keep us in balance. The brain digests a continuous flow of information about the body's position and coordinates compensatory movements. We don't have to think about it: If we stumble to the right, we instinctively arch to the left to keep from falling.

Knowing Where You Stand

Information about your position reaches the brain from three sensory systems:

- ◆ **Somatosensory system:** Receptors on the skin and in the muscles and joints report to the brain. If you've ever tried to walk when your foot has fallen asleep and is temporarily numb, you can appreciate the importance of these receptors.

- ◆ **Vision:** As you might guess if you took the balancing test, the eyes are a very important source of positional information. Try the test again—this time with your eyes open—to see what a difference vision makes.
- ◆ **Vestibular system in the inner ear:** You probably know— perhaps from a bout of dizziness during a severe cold— that fluid-filled canals in the inner ear play a role in balance. As the head moves, this fluid moves, triggering signals from tiny receptor hairs in the canals to the brain.

Why three systems? Each gives only a partial report; the combined information is more complete. Also, redundancy assures that even if one or two of these systems aren't functioning, the message will get through. Of course, it might arrive more slowly and less completely, and the brain would react with reduced speed and coordination.

Staying Upright

Let's see what happens if you have the classic misfortune of slipping on a banana peel. Your somatosensory system would feel your foot fly out from under you; your eyes would observe that your surroundings were moving too quickly; and your vestibular system would sense that you were no longer upright. Whoops! No time to think!

Fortunately, the body is programmed to respond immediately via the nervous system. Your brain sounds the alarm, and an integrated system of reflexes leaps into action, fighting to keep you from falling: Your head and trunk jerk forward; you flail your arms; and the foot that slipped tries to kick itself back to the ground. Thanks to these instinctive efforts, you'd most likely regain your balance.

These dramatic reactions are only part of the story. Your body's balance mechanisms operate constantly. For every step you take, every reach of an arm, every deep breath—any movement that alters, even slightly, your position or center of gravity—your balance reflexes trigger compensatory changes.

BALANCING IN YOUR SLEEP

Your balance system works even if you aren't awake. Have you ever seen someone nod off in a stuffy room? His neck and shoulder muscles relax; his head—no longer supported by these muscles—tips forward and drops toward his chest. Were his head to continue falling, he might lose his balance and tumble out of the chair. But the sudden move stretches his neck extensor muscles, triggering a reflex that snaps his head up again.

BALANCING THROUGH LIFE

Age is just one factor that affects balance, as I'll explain in a minute. While the time line below is accurate for most people, some of us are "young" for our chronological ages while others are "old."

Childhood to teens

Kids have terrific balance. They can run along a fence rail, play hopscotch, and remain vertical as they ride a skateboard around a corner. Young gymnasts perform backward somersaults on balance beams just four inches wide. This incredible ability probably peaks at around age twenty.

Early twenties to early forties

Balance normally remains excellent, not limiting activities in everyday life or even in active sports. A healthy woman can ice skate, ride a bike over bumpy terrain, or run backward with outstretched tennis racket to return a tricky serve—and rarely fall.

Middle forties to early seventies

Experts are just beginning to realize that balance starts to deteriorate in middle age. The changes are so subtle, and arrive so gradually, that they're hard to spot unless you're looking for them. Most women aren't aware of balance problems during these years.

Mid-seventies and older

As small changes mount up, loss of balance begins to affect the quality of life. Active women notice the difference in demanding leisure activities such as biking, skiing, or running. Sedentary women feel less steady when they walk; they slow down, aware that they may fall.

One of the saddest consequences of deteriorating balance, aside from falling itself, is the *fear* of falling. This starts a vicious cycle that diminishes the quality of life. An older person becomes cautious physically—and rightly so. But this can lead to inactivity, weakness, and falls; the falls, in turn, prompt more fear and even less activity.

♦ ♦ ♦

My mother is eighty-five, and last week she had a fall. She was standing and just fell from her full height onto the paved driveway. She scraped her arms and legs, but luckily there was no internal damage or broken bones. Now she has lost her nerve and is timid to go outside. I expect I'll have to move in with her.

> —Letter from a woman who heard me interviewed on the radio

♦ ♦ ♦

WHAT THROWS US OFF BALANCE?

Below are factors that put us at risk for falling. All are cumulative, and many are age-related.

♦ MUSCLE WEAKNESS

Our balancing reflexes can't work unless our muscles are strong and our joints are flexible enough to respond. So it's not surprising that balancing ability is directly related to the strength of our legs and the flexibility of our ankles. That's why strengthening exercises can help significantly.

♦ ♦ ♦

I am sixty-six years old and found myself tripping and falling more frequently. The last fall landed me on my face, splitting a tooth and breaking my glasses! My daughter-in-law suggested I look into your book, which I did. I started off lifting five pounds with my legs and two pounds with my arms. I am now up to twelve pounds on the legs and eight pounds on the arms. I can easily balance on one foot and have had no more falls.
—Thelma

♦ ♦ ♦

♦ AGE-RELATED SENSORY CHANGES

As we get older, the systems that report position to the brain gradually decline: Nerve receptors become less sensitive and vision less clear. We can minimize these changes. For instance, since eyesight is important to good balance—as you know from taking the test at the beginning of this chapter—an accurate eyeglass prescription is an important balancing aid, especially if you wear bifocals.

◆ MEDICAL CONDITIONS

Changes in body and health can affect balance. Here are some examples:

- **Weight gain or loss:** If you've ever been pregnant, you know how extra weight can throw you off balance. Likewise, obese women tend to have poor balance because it's harder for muscles to pull a heavier body back into line. Missing weight can be a problem too: Women who have undergone mastectomies sometimes feel unbalanced if they don't use a weighted prosthesis.
- **Osteoporosis:** Osteoporotic fractures in the vertebrae can cause bent-over posture. This means that the head—which is heavy—is in front of the body instead of perched on top. The lopsided load can impair balance.
- **Neurological disease:** The brain and the nervous system are responsible for maintaining balance. Therefore, balance is impaired by conditions (such as Parkinson's disease) that affect the relevant parts of the brain, the somatosensory system, or balance reflexes.
- **Hypotension:** Low blood pressure—hypotension—can cause dizziness or loss of balance. Normally the body adjusts blood pressure to changes in position. But if a woman has a condition called postural hypotension, her blood pressure may drop precipitously and make her feel dizzy when she stands up or when she moves after standing still for several minutes.

◆ MEDICATIONS

Along with physical problems themselves, medical treatments can affect balance. Among the most common examples are mood-altering or sleep-inducing drugs, medication taken for high blood pressure (which can cause postural hypotension), diuretics, and barbiturates. Doctors may not consider balance when they prescribe, so be aware. If you notice balance problems, ask about adjusting the dose or the timing of the drug, or using a different treatment.

♦ ALCOHOL

Alcohol consumption and abuse are major factors in falls and poor balance. Indeed, loss of balance is such a common effect of drinking that a standard roadside test for sobriety—walking a straight line—is also used in research laboratories to assess balance. Long-term alcohol abuse can damage the brain, thereby affecting balance even when a person isn't drinking. These effects are particularly devastating in the elderly, who start with a balance deficit.

♦ ENVIRONMENTAL HAZARDS

Whether we fall depends not only on how well we can balance but on the challenges thrown at this ability. Environmental hazards—slippery walking surfaces, unseen obstacles such as an appliance cord on the floor—combined with declining balance can cause falls. Remove these problems and the risk is lower. One environmental hazard that's sometimes forgotten: shoes. About half of those who fall are wearing shoes that have unstable heels or that don't provide adequate support.

EXERCISE IMPROVES BALANCE

"Use it or lose it" applies to balance too. We know that physically active people generally have fewer falls (provided they don't take up risky sports such as in-line skating), and that walking and aerobic activity improve coordination and maintain balance. Western scientists are just starting to understand what Eastern medical experts have known for centuries— that yoga, tai chi, and similar activities can improve balance as well as coordination, posture, and flexibility. But this is brand-new territory, and we have so much to learn! For instance, we don't yet fully understand *why* exercise helps; nor do we know how to maximize these benefits.

One of the most exciting results of our *JAMA* study—a finding we never anticipated—was that strength training significantly improves balance. We knew from previous research that muscle strength affects balance, so we included an evaluation in our extensive battery of tests. But we weren't expecting to see much change. After all, our volunteers were middle-aged,

THE FALL-SAFE HOME

You can significantly reduce the risk of falls by eliminating environmental hazards and adding safety features. This is important for all households but especially for those where an elderly person lives or visits.

- Secure rugs to the floor.
- Keep toys and other clutter off the floor.
- Avoid polishes that make floors slippery.
- Wipe up kitchen and bathroom spills promptly.
- Put electrical cords out of the way, so no one trips over them.
- Illuminate stairwells, corridors, and closets, as well as rooms.
- Use night lights or have flashlights readily available.
- Minimize lighting glare, which also impairs good vision.
- Install handrails on both sides of stairwells; put grab bars in the tub and shower.
- Organize cupboards and closets to minimize bending and reaching.

not old. We assumed they were still balancing as well as ever; we figured they didn't have room for improvement. And we were wrong!

To our dismayed surprise, there was an average 8 percent balance decline in the women who didn't strength-train. What happened? They were a year older, for one thing. Another factor, we believe, is that these women became even more sedentary. Meanwhile, the women in our strength-training group showed an average 14 percent *gain* in balance scores. We credit this stunning change in part to their enormous improvements in muscle strength, and in part to the associated neurological changes.

Dorothy, seventy, didn't think she had a balance problem when she started the study. But after a year of strength training, her test score improved by 11 percent—and now she sees the difference.

I'll stand on one foot, put on my sock, and then, since I'm still standing, I'll put on the shoe too. Before I might have gotten one on, but not both. Every so often I'll be standing there, and I'll say to myself, "My goodness, I can do that for quite a while."

As a result of these findings, my strength-training studies now incorporate exercises to improve balance. And I'm delighted to report that other investigators are paying more attention to balance too.

Particularly exciting was a 1997 study by John Campbell and colleagues in New Zealand, which dramatically demonstrated that strength and balance training can reduce falls in the elderly. Over a one-year period, 116 frail women, all age eighty or older, followed a strength-training program similar to the one in this book. In addition, they did special exercises designed to improve their balance, including moves like walking backward and walking on the balls of their feet. Meanwhile, the investigators also observed a control group of similar women who didn't exercise. During the year of the study, the women in the control group had a total of 152 falls. But those who had exercised had only 88 falls—a 53 percent reduction.

I eagerly follow the work of balance-training pioneers like Mary Tinetti, M.D., of the Yale University School of Medicine, and James Judge, M.D., from the University of Connecticut in Farmington. As we learn more, I believe that balance exercises will take their place—along with aerobics, strength training, and flexibility exercises—as physical fitness essentials, especially for older people.

♦ ♦ ♦

Last weekend I was cross-country skiing across a pond. I hit a soft spot, and one leg went down to my knee under the ice. No one could come help me, because they would just go in too. I had to stand on one ski and get my other ski up and out of the

water and then over to the side, because I knew the ice was thin where I was standing. The ski was heavy from all the ice and snow, so the lifting and balancing were very strenuous. I bet I couldn't have done it if my muscles weren't in good shape.
—Charlotte

♦ ♦ ♦

II

GETTING IN GEAR

▼   ▼   ▼   ▼

▼ ▼ ▼ ▼ ▼ ▼ ▼

PREPARING FOR
POSITIVE CHANGE

itness is my profession—and my passion. But I'm also a mom with three young children and a demanding job. Sometimes I'm so over-extended that I just can't find another moment. So even though I know how important exercise is for my health and well-being, and even though I *enjoy* being active, I'm not always as regular about it as I want to be.

My experience makes me very sympathetic to people who have trouble starting a program or keeping up with it. If you're in this category, you have lots of company. By now everyone knows how important it is to exercise. But when researchers go out into the real world and ask people what they're actually doing to stay fit, they find an enormous gap between preaching and practice. True, there are record numbers of gym members, treadmill owners, and triathlon participants. But far more people are sitting on the sidelines. More than three-quarters of American women are sedentary, reports the Centers for Disease Control and Prevention.

Fitness experts used to be impatient with people who just couldn't get moving. These days, most of us in this profession are more realistic. We recognize that it's hard to translate knowledge into action, and we're learning more and more about how to help.

FIVE STAGES OF CHANGE

All of us struggle to make positive changes in our lives—whether it's to quit smoking, keep the desk neat, or begin lifting weights. In the process, we discover that it's quite a challenge to rearrange behavior.

Researchers working with smokers noticed that they moved through certain predictable stages as they tried to quit. At each point they faced different problems and could benefit from different kinds of help. This insight boosted the effectiveness of smoking cessation programs, and it caught the attention of researchers in other fields. It turned out that these stages weren't unique to smoking; people trying to change most behavior went through similar steps. This book was written with these concepts in mind. I'm indebted to James Prochaska, Ph.D., of the University of Rhode Island, who developed the theory, and to Bess Marcus, Ph.D., from Brown University, who adapted the ideas to exercise.

Here are the five stages you'll pass through as you make strength training part of your life:

> **Stage 1: Precontemplation:** You don't know about strength training; you don't realize what it can do for you. Therefore, you don't see a need for it and don't have any desire to do it.
>
> **Stage 2: Contemplation:** You've become interested in strength training; you know it will make you stronger and healthier. You want to start a program—but don't know where to begin.
>
> **Stage 3: Preparation:** You're not lifting weights yet. But you've moved past merely thinking about it and are taking concrete steps to get ready.
>
> **Stage 4: Action:** This is an exciting stage—the first six months of a strength-training program. You're making progress, enjoying the exercises, seeing benefits.
>
> **Stage 5: Maintenance:** The program has become a routine part of your life—a habit you wouldn't think of breaking, just like brushing your teeth.

Some people move smoothly through these five stages. They learn about strength training and decide to try it. They quickly buy the weights, set aside time to do the exercises, and make a start. A year later they're stronger and leaner and committed to the program.

A good example is Mimi, who e-mailed this enthusiastic report:

I have been an avid walker for over twenty years but did not feel strong, especially in my upper body. I read a review of Strong Women Stay Young *in* Walking *magazine and bought the book. I started with three- to five-pound weights and became hooked immediately. At the end of six months I was up to twenty pounds for legs and ten to fifteen pounds for arms. I had more energy and could not believe the changes in my body. I have gone from size 12 jeans to size 8; my "love handles" are gone. My eighteen- and twenty-one-year-old athletic children say, "Gosh, Mom," when I flex my muscles. People constantly say, "You've lost weight," even though I really haven't. I have been doing this for thirteen months now, and I love the way I feel.*

I hope all this happens to you! Indeed, you may be well into the process already. Perhaps you bought weights along with this book. Or maybe you've been training for some time and are now looking for a more systematic program to follow.

For other women, the path is a little rockier; their hopes don't readily translate into action. If you're in this situation, this chapter can help.

STAGE 1: PRECONTEMPLATION

It doesn't take much effort to leave the precontemplation stage—in fact, if you're reading this book, you're already past it. Usually, all that's needed is some information. Once you're aware that strength training has significant health benefits and are beginning to think about doing it, you're at Stage 2.

What if a friend or relative is at the precontemplation stage and you'd like to get her started? You could suggest she read the first four chapters of this book so she'll understand just how much strength training could do for her.

STAGE 2: CONTEMPLATION

I meet many people who are in the contemplation stage. They're excited about lifting weights, they want to get started—but they don't know exactly how. Some women get the information and run with it. That's what happened with Lisa. She had been reading about strength training, and then she had this experience:

> I was taking a canoeing class with about fourteen people, and that day we were going solo. Each of us had to get into a canoe from the dock. Usually I was very careful to hold on and keep my weight low, but this time I just stepped in. The canoe slid out from under me and I fell into the Charles River.
>
> The instructor said, "This is an excellent opportunity to demonstrate how we get back into a canoe if we fall out." I was standing in water up to my shoulders; the instructor was holding my canoe—and now I had to haul myself into it. There was no way. I pulled and kicked for what seemed like hours, but I just didn't have the strength in my upper arms. It was so humiliating. The whole canoeing class was watching from the water; a kayaking class and boathouse attendants were watching from the dock. Finally, the instructor got out of his canoe, went onto the dock, and he and one of the boathouse attendants grabbed my arms and hauled me out.
>
> I was perfectly safe the whole time, but I thought, what if I'd really needed to do this and I couldn't? I started strength training soon afterward.

Other women think about exercising, only to let the idea slip away. Jayne read about my research in the *Tufts University Health & Nutrition Letter* and contacted me for more information. She told me she'd always been sedentary but knew she needed to exercise. Jayne recalls:

The exercises sounded tolerable—I liked the idea of something that was only twice a week, that I could do without changing clothes or leaving my house, and that didn't involve sweating or lying on the floor. So I decided to try them. I got the information in March. Six months later, I still hadn't done anything about it.

Tap Your Motivations

When I work with a woman like Jayne, who was stuck at the contemplation stage, I start by tapping her motivations. I ask her to write down all the reasons she wants to exercise. Not everyone needs to do this. But if you've spent weeks or months at the contemplation stage, you've learned that just *thinking* about your motivations isn't enough. In that case I urge you to write them down or describe them to a friend. Taking this simple step is very important: It moves you out of inactive mode and into action.

Here's what Jayne wrote:

1. *I'm only forty-three, but I'm starting to feel creaky. I've never been fit, but I always could get away with it—now I can't and I know I really need to do something. This seems like a good place to begin. I would like to do aerobics at some point, and it would be easier if I'm stronger.*

2. *My knees hurt, and my doctor said that strengthening exercises might help.*

3. *I love the idea that having more muscles will let me eat a little more without gaining weight.*

Nearly thirty years ago, Gerald Kenyon, M.D., of the Royal Surrey Hospital in London, outlined six reasons that motivate people to exercise. They're just as valid today. Have a look at the list—it may expand your thinking. The point is to focus on your reasons for starting this program, whatever they may be. This will get you started and help you stick with it.

♦ Enjoyment of the Activity Itself

I love to lift weights. I relish the challenge of seeing how much I can do; I like the feeling afterward when my muscles are warm and relaxed. Enjoyment may be low on your list of reasons to exercise. However, after you've been doing it for a while, you may surprise yourself.

♦ Health and Fitness Benefits

If you've read the first four chapters of this book, you know that strength training offers impressive health benefits. So even if you don't like exercise, think of it as a means toward an important end.

Ursula was prompted to begin strengthening exercises by changes in her body as she approached her fiftieth birthday:

> I'd never focused on caring for my body; I just assumed it was supposed to work. But I didn't feel as strong anymore. I had always enjoyed physical activities—such as working in the garden and building things with my husband. I could still do them, but it was becoming much more strenuous. I would get out of breath; I'd have to work more slowly; I would feel it more afterward.
>
> Menopause was coming up, with the issue of hormone replacement therapy, and I hadn't sorted it out yet. I was trying to figure out what one might do instead to deal with brittle bones.

Dorothy was one of the participants in our research on strength training. She recalls:

> I have eleven children and seventeen grandchildren. I used to get depressed thinking, "I'll be gone when I'm seventy-five or eighty, and I won't see my grandchildren grow up." Now I have confidence that I'll be around for a long time.

♦ Improvements in Appearance

Strength training can make a big difference in how you look. It tones your body—decreases fat and increases muscle—and improves the way you carry yourself.

Verna, another of our research volunteers, comments:

My weight wasn't out of control before I started, but my arms and inner thighs were flabby, and I was developing quite a tummy. The exercises tightened everything up. I didn't think I could do that after four children.

♦ Social Opportunities

Exercise can be very rewarding socially. I've met some of my best friends through sports. And it's also been the way I keep up with friends who share this interest—and who, like me, don't have much time for socializing. My closest friend from graduate school is an athlete. In the summer we hike together; in the winter we go cross-country skiing. We get a chance to talk, and meanwhile we're doing something physical that we both enjoy.

♦ Stress Reduction and Emotional Well-Being

Exercise is a great way to lift your mood. Research shows that both strengthening and aerobic workouts release tension and decrease depression. Readers often describe emotional benefits. Peg wrote:

At age thirty-three, I'd grown sick of feeling dumpy and washed up. From day one of the weight training, I noticed a drastic improvement in my posture and self-confidence. I now walk tall and proud—for the first time in about eight years.

I find that a strength-training session leaves me feeling de-stressed and energized—this feeling begins an hour or two after the session and lasts through the next day. Research suggests it's a typical reaction.

♦ Thrill Seeking

Mountain climbing and downhill skiing are thrilling experiences—I know, because I enjoy both. But it's also thrilling to set personal goals and see results. Fifteen years ago, when I was single and still in graduate school, my fitness goal was to run a three-hour marathon—and it was very exciting to come within two minutes of that. My life and priorities are different now, but I'm still goal-oriented, and that's one of the reasons I enjoy strength training. It makes me feel good about myself to get stronger. And indirectly, it's responsible for continuing thrills from mountain climbing and skiing—staying strong allows me to participate in these demanding activities, even though I do them infrequently.

Eliminate the Obstacles

When a woman has trouble starting, I urge her to assume she *will* start. Our next task is to figure out exactly what's holding her back and to address the barriers one by one.

Jayne was embarrassed to tell me her list of obstacles:

> *There's no good reason. I could say I'm too busy—and I really am busy—but I manage to find time for other things, like watching the news and reading magazines. I'm tired. I guess what it boils down to is that I'm lazy.*

Actually, Jayne was echoing the reasons—busy, tired, lazy—that turned up in a survey of 1,018 inactive Americans conducted by the President's Council on Physical Fitness and Sports. So let's tackle them, along with other common problems:

♦ "I'm Too Busy; I Don't Have Time."

This is my number-one barrier, and it's what I hear most often from other women. It's not just an excuse—it's a reality.

When I work with someone who's incredibly busy, I ask her to tell me what she does every day during the week. And we try to figure out where she could slip in two strength-training sessions. Here are some possibilities:

- Exercise before work or during lunch hour. This is what I often do with colleagues. I don't need to change clothes, as I would if I did aerobics.
- Schedule workouts to coincide with a TV program, so you have a little fun while you do something for your body.

- Make a date with a friend or family member. You'll get through the exercises. And meanwhile, you'll spend time with someone you like.
- Divide the program into two parts and do four short sessions each week. For instance, you could do the arm exercises one day and the leg exercises the next.
- Get up earlier two mornings a week.
- Take a hard look at your schedule. Often something else is lower priority and can be cut. Or maybe you can shift a responsibility to someone else.

◆ "I'M TOO TIRED—I JUST DON'T HAVE THE ENERGY."

If you can just start, you'll wind up with *more* energy as a result. In the beginning, though, you may have to do the exercises despite fatigue, difficult as that is. Try to focus your attention away from how tired you are and onto the reasons you want to do the program. A written list can be very helpful.

◆ "I'M LAZY; I DON'T HAVE THE WILLPOWER."

Hearing this always makes me sad. Often it means that a woman doesn't feel good about herself. Exercise not only isn't enjoyable for her, it's a source of guilt and unhappiness.

Don't waste energy putting yourself down. Think positively about the benefits you can gain from strength training and why they're important to you. Then congratulate yourself for moving into the contemplation stage.

◆ "I'M TOO OLD" OR "I'M TOO OUT OF SHAPE TO LIFT WEIGHTS."

People in their nineties do these exercises. You're probably in better shape than they were when they began! Nevertheless, you should discuss any concerns with your doctor before you start.

◆ "It's Too Expensive."

Yes, you will have to use equipment to do this program, and you'll probably have to pay for it. For some people, this is a significant issue. But as I'll explain in Chapter 6, you can minimize costs by sharing weights with friends; also, you don't have to buy everything at once. If you want to work out on machines, you may have access to strength-training equipment at your place of employment, or you could join a Y or community center.

I sometimes hear complaints about cost from women who manage to afford luxuries such as expensive makeup or a night at the theater. And I can't help thinking that for the same money they spend on a single splurge, they could buy all the strength-training equipment they'd need for their entire lives.

STAGE 3: PREPARATION

You want to begin; you're eager to learn how to proceed. This book provides all that information. During the preparation stage, you'll buy equipment, you'll read the chapters that describe the exercises, and you'll figure out when and where you're going to do them. Then you'll be ready for the next step—action.

Jayne bought the weights. But then she got stuck again:

I bought the weights and went through the exercises later the same day, just to try them out. Things got hectic at work and I didn't work out again that week. The next week I was off on a trip. When I got back, I decided to ask some friends if they'd do the program with me, but somehow I never got around to calling them. So there was this bag of unused weights sitting in my bedroom closet. And it was very depressing.

I suggest you give yourself a time limit for accomplishing the preliminary tasks. This may sound unnecessary—and indeed, some people don't need a deadline. But I recommend it for everybody because it's such a simple and effective way to move forward. If you run into stumbling blocks, the best antidote is to sit down with a pencil, your calendar, and a notepad, and do the following:

- Make a list of the equipment you need (see Chapter 6).
- Get out the Yellow Pages, look under "Sporting Goods," and write down places to shop. Plan a time to buy the equipment, and put it on your calendar.
- Check your schedule. Decide what days of the week and what times you want to do the exercises. Write the appointments on your calendar. This really helps.
- If you want to train with a friend, figure out when you're going to call and write it on your calendar.
- Make any necessary arrangements to clear your workout times. For instance, if you need to discuss child care with your husband, give yourself a deadline for doing it.
- Finally, of course, keep all the appointments!

Writing down a list of specific tasks is such a simple thing to do. But over the years I've been amazed by its powerful effect. People who'd been struggling to start suddenly begin working their way down their list.

STAGE 4: ACTION

You've bought the equipment and fixed a time to do the exercises. Now you *can't wait* for your first session! The action stage is particularly exciting: You're doing something new, you're enjoying it, and you like the changes you see in yourself. Chapter 10, "Staying on Track," has many suggestions to help you when you reach this point. If you can stick with the program through the critical first six months, you graduate to the next stage—maintenance. By the time the first edition of this book was published, Jayne was on her way:

I'm finally doing it. I recruited a couple of friends to work out with me—women I like, whom I wanted to see more often. We meet at my house every Monday, before dinner, which is a good time to tuck it in. It's helpful to have the regular appointment, and socializing makes the exercise more fun.

God knows I'm not perfect. I rarely miss the session with my friends. But I'm not as reliable about the second session, the one I do myself. And when I'm out of town, forget it. Still, I get going again when I'm back home. It really is becoming part of my life.

Two and a half years later, the group has disbanded. But most of the women—including Jayne—still strength-train. Says Jayne, "It's a miracle!"

STAGE 5: MAINTENANCE

This is the stage where strength training has become a habit and you see lifelong benefits to your health and well-being. But the women I work with don't continue strength training just because it's a habit. They feel an incredible sense of empowerment and spiritual well-being. They've accomplished something important for themselves. They look better and feel better than they have for years. And because of all this, they really don't want to stop.

Dorothy—the grandmother of seventeen whom I quoted earlier in this chapter—joined a YMCA to continue strength training after our study was finished. She added new strengthening exercises to her workouts and she power-walks for three miles every other day. To warm up for her workouts at the Y, she shoots baskets on their basketball court. Says Dorothy (who is now seventy-one):

My children enjoy bragging about me. Their friends are always asking them, "Gee, what does your mom do to stay so healthy and look so good?" This helps keep me going!

I have to keep reminding myself I'm not in my fifties. People are always surprised by my age—not only because I look younger but because I walk briskly and do so much. I have the energy and confidence to try physical things.

Three summers ago Dorothy joined her son and grandchildren for a Wyoming vacation that included horseback riding and white water river-rafting. The following year, she parasailed in Hawaii—soaring nine hundred feet above the water, relishing a glorious view of the mountains of Maui, while her sister watched from the shore with amazement. And last year, back in Hawaii with her cousins, she hopped on a surfboard and rode the waves. Dorothy's latest accomplishment? This year she worked with a fitness instructor at the Y to prepare for the Senior Olympics—and she won a silver medal! I can't wait to hear what she does next.

EQUIPPED FOR
ACTION

T he weekend before I wrote this chapter, I stacked a cord of wood. Isn't a physically demanding activity like this just as good as strength training with dumbbells? Surprisingly, it's not. Stacking the wood was quite a challenge, but my muscles didn't have to work as hard with each lift as they do in a strength-training session. Picking up larger armloads of wood might have given my biceps a better workout, but the awkward position could have strained my back. And obviously, this isn't something I can readily do twice a week.

Using equipment lets you strengthen your muscles safely and systematically. The women in my study worked out on strength-training machines in our laboratory at Tufts. You can find similar machines at many fitness centers—and if you have a spare room and money isn't an issue, you can purchase versions for your home. But you don't need to join a gym or buy costly weight machines. You can get the same benefits from a strength-training program done at home with inexpensive equipment. All you will ever need are the following:

- Ankle weights
- Dumbbells
- A container to store the weights
- A sturdy chair
- A towel
- Comfortable clothes

DOING THE PROGRAM WITH FREE WEIGHTS

Free weights are weights that you hold in your hand or strap to your body—in contrast to weights that are part of a machine. This is the least expensive type of strength-training equipment, but it's definitely *not* second best. Indeed, many professional bodybuilders prefer free weights because of their versatility.

You can start this program with free weights—ankle weights and dumbbells—that cost around $120. Later, as you get stronger, you'll need to spend another $20 to $50 for heavier dumbbells. If you think about it, $140 to $170 really isn't very much for equipment that never breaks down or wears out.

Ankle Weights

Three of the leg exercises in the basic program, as well as several of the supplemental exercises in Chapter 11, use ankle weights. These are strap-on cuffs with compartments for up to twenty pounds of weighted bars. You adjust the weight of the cuff by adding or removing these bars.

In the beginning, you'll work out with three to five pounds in each cuff, depending on your present strength. If you're like most women, you'll probably double the load during the first twelve weeks of the program, and by the end of six months, you'll be lifting ten to twenty pounds with each leg. So you'll need two ankle cuffs, each holding up to twenty pounds.

Several companies make satisfactory cuffs; the two top brands are All Pro and Keiser. Twenty-pound leg weights cost about $40 to $50 each. When you shop, you may be tempted to get ten-pound cuffs, since they're a lot less expensive—but I don't recommend it. Since you'll almost certainly need heavier weights to keep progressing, it's cheaper in the long run to purchase the twenty-pound versions right away. I sometimes provide very frail, elderly women with ten-pound ankle cuffs because they can barely lift two pounds at the start. But these women often surprise me by graduating to larger cuffs six months later.

♦ ♦ ♦

The salesman in the sporting goods store thought I was crazy to buy twenty-pound ankle weights. But I've been adding a pound a week and I think I'll fill those babies up. Maybe I'll go back to the store and kick him!
—Valerie (who's just kidding)

♦ ♦ ♦

A money-saving option is to buy just one ankle weight. Instead of al-ternating legs as you do the exercises, complete two sets of each exercise on one leg, then move the weight to the other leg and do another two sets. This works, but it's less convenient. Also, it puts additional strain on the sup-porting leg for those exercises done standing. If you decide to work with a single ankle weight, make sure you don't lock the knee of your supporting leg, since that increases stress on the joint. And if you experience knee pain in the supporting leg, consider investing in a second ankle weight.

Dumbbells

During the first week you'll be doing the arm exercises with dumbbells that weigh from one to three pounds. But most women triple this by their twelfth week of strength training and eventually go past ten pounds for most of the arm exercises.

Dumbbells can be purchased in one-pound increments, all the way from one pound up to fifteen or twenty pounds, which is as much as you're likely to need. A complete set is very handy, but it would be expensive. Also, twenty pairs of dumbbells would take up a lot of space. Here's my sugges-tion for a workable compromise between convenience and cost:

- ◆ Instead of buying dumbbells in one-, two-, three-, or four-pound sizes—which you'll outgrow after one or two sessions—use the weighted bars from your ankle cuffs. This is not particularly glamorous, but it's economical. When you're using two bars, tape them together securely with at least three rounds of silver duct tape. Don't try to go above four pounds, though; the bundle will be too big for your hands.
- ◆ Buy pairs of five-, eight-, and ten-pound dumbbells when you start the program. For most women, these will suffice for several months.
- ◆ Assess your needs again when you graduate to the ten-pound dumbbells and are looking ahead. At this point

you may want pairs of twelve-pound and perhaps also fifteen-pound or even twenty-pound dumbbells.

Here are other ways to cut costs.

◆ Buy Adjustable Dumbbells

These sets may be cheaper than dumbbells bought separately, though not necessarily. Make sure they can be adjusted quickly, because you'll probably need to change the amount of weight from exercise to exercise. Also check that they're balanced evenly at every weight, so they won't be awkward to use.

◆ Share Weights

Maybe a friend or neighbor is interested in doing the program. If you're working out with other people, it's easy to share—since each individual progresses at her own rate, you're likely to reach different levels at different times.

◆ Buy Used Dumbbells

Check the classified ads in your local newspaper or look in the Yellow Pages for a shop that sells used sporting goods. You can sell dumbbells you've outgrown the same way.

Container for the Weights

For safety's sake, keep weights in a container unless they're actually being lifted. I store my equipment in two strong canvas tote bags: The bags hold up well, and they have handles that make them easy to move. One bag would suffice if I didn't have to move the weights around.

Other possibilities:

- Duffel bag
- Sturdy box or carton (more difficult to move)
- Strong wicker baskets (attractive, but may not last as long)
- Rack designed to hold weights (harder to move; not safe if small children have access to it)

Chair

You'll do some of the exercises while seated in a chair; for others you'll stand and hold on to the back. Find the chair in your house that's best suited to the job—often a dining room chair is just right. If you're not sure, experiment with different chairs and see which you prefer. Here's what you're looking for:

- Strong and stable construction
- No arms
- Seat high and deep enough so that when you sit all the way back in the chair, your feet barely touch the ground and your knee joint is just over the edge of the seat. Obviously this is easier for shorter women than for taller women.
- Chair back high enough so you can stand behind it and hold on for balance without bending over.

Towel

One of the leg exercises is done seated with a rolled-up towel under your knees; the towel pads the underside of your legs and keeps them in the correct position. Pick a spare bath towel you can keep with your weights so you don't have to look for it each time you work out.

What to Wear

You don't need special clothing for this program—in fact, some women do the exercises at the office in their work clothes. However, I recommend the following for comfort:

- ◆ Loose clothing made from cotton or other breathable fabric so you don't get hot
- ◆ Thick socks or leg warmers to prevent the ankle weights from chafing
- ◆ Sturdy, supportive shoes that have a sole flexible enough for you to stand on your toes. Sneakers or athletic shoes are fine; however, firm leather-soled shoes won't give you the necessary flexibility, and light sneakers or canvas shoes don't have adequate support.

Where Can I Buy the Weights?

Dumbbells up to ten pounds are widely available. These days you'll find them in discount and department stores, as well as in shops that sell sporting equipment. But for heavier dumbbells and for ankle cuffs, you'll probably need a specialty store. Check the Yellow Pages under "Sporting Goods" to find places near you, and call to make sure they have what you need.

Many women prefer to order their weights by mail, not only for shopping convenience but to avoid transporting them home. Just remember that heavy shipping weights can be costly. Here are sources:

ALL PRO EXERCISE PRODUCTS, INC.
P.O. Box 8268
Longboat Key, FL 34228
Tel: 1-800-735-9287
Fax: 1-941-387-7901
http://www.allproweights.com

MC SPORTS
3070 Shaffer Street, S.E.
Grand Rapids, MI 49512
Tel: 1-800-626-1762 or
1-616-942-2600
Fax: 1-616-942-1973

KEISER SPORTS HEALTH EQUIPMENT
2470 South Cherry Avenue
Fresno, CA 93706
Tel: 1-800-888-7009
1-559-256-8000
Fax: 1-559-256-8100

PARAGON SPORTING GOODS
867 Broadway
New York, NY 10003
Tel: 1-212-255-8036
Fax: 1-212-929-1831

Keiserinstitute on aging. Com

FITNESS DISTRIBUTORS
17 South Avenue
Natick, MA 01760
Tel: 1-800-244-1882 or
1-508-653-1882
Fax: 1-508-650-0448

99.90
30, 31
130, 21
info
 # cust #497-1248

FITNESS FIRST
P.O. Box 251
Shawnee Mission, KS 66201
Tel: 1-800-421-1791 or
1-913-384-6262
Fax: 1-800-421-0036
http://www.fitness1st.com

COUNTRY TECHNOLOGY, INC.
P.O. Box 87
Gays Mills, WI 54631
Tel: 1-608-735-4718
Fax: 1-608-735-4859

One brand of adjustable dumbbells is Intellbell's PowerBlock. For information, contact the company:

1819 South Cedar Avenue
Owatonna, MN 55060
Tel: 1-800-446-5215 or
1-507-451-5152
http://www.powerblock.com

HOME GYM EQUIPMENT

The equipment described above is all you need to do this program. I'm often asked about another option, home strength-training machines. These are considerably more costly—you can expect to spend $500 to $4,000—and require a great deal more space. Also, you may need assistance from a personal trainer to adapt the instructions in this book to the particular equipment you purchase.

Home gym equipment ranges from a simple bench with attachments for arm and leg exercises (around $500) to complicated room-size multistation machines ($1,000 to $4,000 and up). There are many options, and new models come out all the time, so I can't comment on each one, but I'll give you some general pointers.

Some multistation machines use thick bands instead of weights. Although this type of system can be beneficial, I prefer home machines with weight stacks—I find them easier to use, and they don't limit the range of motion through which you do the exercise. That's important, because doing the full movement improves your flexibility. Some machines use your body weight for resistance, which can work well.

If you decide to buy a strength-training machine, I suggest you go to a store that specializes in sporting goods. Look for a place that offers several brands, not just one, and whose sales staff is knowledgeable about the equipment. Here are questions to ask:

- **Which muscle groups can I train with this equipment?** Ask the salesperson to demonstrate the exercises and try them yourself.
- **Will this equipment fit me?** Before you buy a home gym, make sure it's comfortable for you. This is especially important for petite women. Most home gyms are still made for larger, taller men, though this is changing. Still, the shorter you are, the more difficult it will be to find equipment that fits your body.
- **Can I adjust the equipment by myself?** Don't just watch the salesperson make the adjustments—see if they're easy for you to do.

- **How much space does the machine require?** Equipment looks smaller in a store than it will in your home. Some strength-training machines fill an entire room.
- **How long is the warranty? If I needed a repair, what would I do?**

OTHER EQUIPMENT

One reason this program is so safe and effective is that you can accurately monitor your progress. Because you know exactly how much weight you're lifting, you can decide when you need to continue at the same level and when it's time to move forward. But women often ask me about other kinds of strength-training equipment.

◆ CAN I USE EXERCISE BANDS?

These are wide rubber bands that usually come in color-coded sets of varying thicknesses that make them harder or easier to pull. They're cheap, and they don't weigh very much. But bands have drawbacks as well:

- They need to be anchored properly, which makes them harder to use than free weights.
- You don't know how much resistance you're pulling against, so it's not as easy to track your progress.
- Most people rapidly progress to the highest level and remain at that point even though they have the physical capacity to get stronger.
- As the band stretches, the resistance increases—unlike weights, which remain constant through the entire move. Greater resistance can prevent you from going through the full range of motion when you do an exercise, so you might not see the improvements in flexibility you can expect from a strengthening program.

Many people enjoy the bands, though, and they can be beneficial if used appropriately. Some women who normally work out with free weights tuck a band into a suitcase if they're traveling—they couldn't do that as easily with a pair of ankle cuffs and two ten-pound dumbbells!

♦ What About Homemade Equipment?

I've seen suggestions ranging from lifting one-pound soup cans (harmless for you and the soup, but it won't build muscle), to lifting buckets or gallon jugs filled with sand or gravel (potentially dangerous).

Please don't improvise this way! Plastic jugs and buckets are not made for strength training: They're not manufactured to hold that much weight; the handles are designed for carrying, not for the kind of lifting done in this program. They could break and even injure you. Similarly, do-it-yourself ankle weights are risky.

You're about to start a program that will require your time—the most valuable thing you have, if you think about it. I urge you to do justice to your efforts and buy the appropriate equipment. This is the first step in a commitment to improving your health and well-being, not just now but for the rest of your life.

III

THE STRONG WOMEN STAY YOUNG PROGRAM

▼　▼　▼　▼

STRENGTH-
TRAINING BASICS
FOR SAFE
WORKOUTS

Y ou've assembled your equipment: weights (and a storage container for
them), a sturdy chair, and a towel. You're wearing comfortable clothes,
supportive shoes, and thick socks. And now you're ready to learn the
exercises. But before that, a few preliminaries.

First, I'd like you to take a simple test. It's called the PAR-Q—Physical Activity Readiness Questionnaire. You may have seen it before, because
it's widely used. PAR-Q was developed by the Canadian Society for Exercise
Physiology to quickly tell you if you can start an exercise program immediately or if you should see your doctor first. If you have health concerns, also
look at the box on page 149 before you begin.

PAR-Q & YOU

(A Questionnaire for People Aged 15 to 69)

Regular physical activity is fun and healthy, and increasingly more people are starting to become more active every day. Being more active is very safe for most people. However, some people should check with their doctor before they start becoming much more physically active.

If you are planning to become much more physically active than you are now, start by answering the seven questions in the box below. If you are between the ages of 15 and 69, the PAR-Q will tell you if you should check with your doctor before you start. If you are over 69 years of age and you are not used to being very active, check with your doctor.

Common sense is your best guide when you answer these questions. Please read the questions carefully and answer each one honestly: check YES or NO.

YES NO

☐   ☐   1. Has your doctor ever said that you have a heart condition <u>and</u> that you should only do physical activity recommended by a doctor?

☐   ☐   2. Do you feel pain in your chest when you do physical activity?

☐   ☐   3. In the past month, have you had chest pain when you were not doing physical activity?

☐   ☐   4. Do you lose your balance because of dizziness or do you ever lose consciousness?

☐   ☐   5. Do you have a bone or joint problem that could be made worse by a change in your physical activity?

☐   ☐   6. Is your doctor currently prescribing drugs (for example, water pills) for your blood pressure or heart condition?

☐   ☐   7. Do you know of <u>any other reason</u> why you should not do physical activity?

IF YOU ANSWERED

YES to one or more questions

Talk with your doctor by phone or in person BEFORE you start becoming much more physically active or BEFORE you have a fitness appraisal. Tell your doctor about the PAR-Q and which questions you answered YES.

- You may be able to do any activity you want—as long as you start slowly and build up gradually. Or, you may need to restrict your activities to those which are safe for you. Talk with your doctor about the kinds of physical activities you wish to participate in, and follow his/her advice.
- Find out which community programs are safe and helpful for you.

NO to all questions

If you answered NO honestly to *all* PAR-Q questions, you can be reasonably sure that you can:

- start becoming much more physically active—begin slowly and build up gradually. This is the safest and easiest way to go.
- take part in a fitness appraisal—this is an excellent way to determine your basic fitness so that you can plan the best way for you to live actively.

DELAY BECOMING MUCH MORE ACTIVE:

- if you are not feeling well because of a temporary illness such as a cold or fever—wait until you feel better; or
- if you are or may be pregnant—talk to your doctor before you start becoming more active.

Please note: If your health changes so that you then answer YES to any of the above questions, tell your fitness or health professional. Ask whether you should change your physical activity plan.

Informed Use of the PAR-Q: The Canadian Society for Exercise Physiology, Health Canada, and their agents assume no liability for persons who undertake physical activity, and if in doubt after completing this questionnaire, consult your doctor prior to physical activity.

SAFETY COMES FIRST

Strength training carries less risk of injury than many other physical activities, including jogging and aerobics. It's safe for nearly everyone—our research subjects have ranged from Olympic medalists to frail ninety-year-olds. Because we place so much emphasis on safety, injuries have been rare.

You'll prevent problems by heeding the simple precautions below. And you'll also have more effective workouts.

Create an Area for Training

This program requires very little space—just enough for a chair, plus room around it on all sides to allow free movement. Clear this small area of other furniture, loose rugs, toys, electrical cords, and other hazards. I don't normally think of kids and pets as "hazards"—I have three children, two cats, and a dog. But when I'm training, I make sure they're not around the equipment.

Several exercises call for a sturdy chair to help you balance yourself. If possible, place the chair on a secure carpet, so it doesn't slide along the floor. An alternative, if you have bare floors, is to stabilize the chair by putting it against a wall.

Keep Your Weights in a Container

During a workout, only the dumbbells or leg weights you're actually using should be out of the container. *As soon as you finish an exercise, stow the weight!* Make this a habit right from the start instead of learning the hard way, as I did. When my daughter Alexandra was two, she grabbed a five-pound dumbbell that I'd carelessly left on a counter within her reach. That dumbbell hadn't seemed very heavy or dangerous—until she pulled it off the counter and it fell on her toes. No bones were broken, fortunately, but it was a painful experience for both of us.

BACK SAFETY TIPS

If you have a bad back, I know you'll be careful when you perform the exercises. But it's also important to pamper your back when you transport your equipment.

- If possible, store your weights next to the chair in your workout area, so you don't have to move them for each session. If you must keep them elsewhere, move them carefully.
- Don't lift too much at once when you're carrying the weights. Make several trips if necessary.
- Lift the container properly: Bend at the knees, and rise slowly.
- Sit down to put on the leg weights. Rest your feet on a stool or coffee table to make it easier.
- After exercising, take similar precautions when you remove the weights and stow them.

Don't Walk Around with Your Leg Weights On

Your ankle weights may not feel very heavy, but they affect walking. You may feel steady on your feet when you're wearing them, but

- the unaccustomed weight could throw you off balance,
- the fastening straps may snag on each other, and
- your ability to recover from tripping could be impaired.

So why take chances?

Plan ahead to avoid interruptions that would require you to walk during a training session.

- **Children:** Make sure youngsters stay safely away from your weights while you're exercising. Or strength-train when the kids are asleep, out of the house, or under someone else's supervision.
- **Doorbell:** Ask another household member to respond, or put a sign on the door to explain that you're busy.
- **Telephone:** Have someone else monitor the phone or let the answering machine take calls; move the telephone to a nearby table so you can reach it during your workout.

If something urgent comes up, *stop to remove your leg weights before you leave your workout space.*

Take the Day Off If You're Tired or Aren't Feeling Well

You won't lose anything by skipping a day occasionally. And there's little to gain by exercising when you're too exhausted or sick to do your best. Give yourself a break, get better—and then resume your workouts.

Get Enough to Drink

Strength training doesn't make you sweat, so it doesn't increase your need for liquids the way aerobic exercise does. Nevertheless, it's wise to have a drink before you start and to keep a beverage within easy reach so you don't have to leave the workout area if you get thirsty. What should you drink? Water is fine; you can drink a sports beverage if you prefer the taste, but it's not necessary.

Many people, especially as they get older, don't drink enough fluid, and they're often underhydrated. This makes it easy for them to become de-hydrated if they get sick or the weather turns hot. Regardless of your age, try to drink eight glasses of liquid a day. This may sound like a lot, but it's not hard to consume that much if you have one or two glasses with each meal, and drink between meals when possible.

And speaking of drinking: Even a small amount of alcohol—as little as one glass of wine or beer—slows your reaction time. So if you've had a drink, wait a couple of hours before you do these exercises.

Work Out Between Meals

It's best to be neither very hungry nor very full when you strength-train. If you're very hungry, exertion could make you light-headed or dizzy. And right after a heavy meal, a lot of your blood goes to your digestive tract. A workout will be less taxing if you wait an hour or two.

Maintain Good Posture

As you learn each exercise, check that your posture matches the illustration on the next page. Proper posture helps avoid muscle strain and injury, not only during workouts but in everyday life—and keeps you looking young.

Good posture doesn't mean the stiff stance of a Marine at attention. Your body should be relaxed but standing tall. The same applies to good seated posture: Sit tall in the chair. Your legs should be at a 90-degree angle to your torso, with your feet touching the floor. Check yourself in a mirror, or ask a friend to check you. Here's a good posture trick that trainers suggest: Imagine someone has attached a string to the top of your head and is gently pulling it up.

Check your posture:
- ◆ Chin is tipped in, to be in line with the neck
- ◆ Neck is in line with the spine
- ◆ Shoulders are back, down, and relaxed
- ◆ Back is straight
- ◆ Pelvis is slightly tucked under
- ◆ Knees are neither locked nor bent

Relax

When we contract one muscle, we have a tendency to tense others as well. This can be helpful in real life—for instance, if you're struggling to lift a heavy suitcase, your biceps may need an assist from muscles in your shoulders and back. But during strength training, only the muscles you're working should contract. First, you want these muscles to get a full workout. But even more important, tensing your entire body contributes to stress. If you relax, you will feel more peaceful and the exercises will be more enjoyable.

Try to identify your tension tendencies so you can correct them. For instance, when I lift weights, I have a tendency to scrunch my shoulders up around my ears. And if I'm not careful, I clench my teeth. During a workout, I need to consciously relax my jaw and shoulders.

Move Slowly

I want to emphasize how important it is—for safety and for optimal results—to do the exercises slowly. Unless you make an effort to pace yourself, you will most likely perform the lifts too quickly—or speed up as a session continues. One reason is that speed can enhance strength in everyday life. For instance, a way to lift a very heavy suitcase is to swing it. This is a common cause of back, shoulder, or hip injuries—as you may know from painful experience. What's more, muscles won't get trained if momentum (or gravity) moves the weight. Slow, smooth moves recruit more motor units and involve more muscle fibers in the lift, which means that the entire muscle benefits.

Keep Breathing!

You might not think you need a reminder to breathe, but believe it or not, most people forget. This happens out of habit, because it's yet another instinctive trick we use to boost strength slightly in everyday life. Holding your breath creates pressure in the chest and abdominal cavity, which prevents blood from leaving the muscles. Professional weight lifters use this technique—it's called the Valsalva maneuver—to give themselves an edge. That's why they grunt (the sound comes from the glottis, the opening between the vocal cords, closing and cutting off air) and why veins bulge in their necks and heads. This could be dangerous, especially for someone with a condition—such as heart disease, diabetes, or glaucoma—that makes the blood vessels vulnerable.

After a Vacation or Illness

If you need to put the program on hold for two or more weeks, don't expect to resume at the same level as before. Reduce the amount you lift, just to be on the safe side. Then gradually increase the weight again as your muscles readjust.

After I warn people not to hold their breath when they lift a weight, they sometimes go to the other extreme and hyperventilate. Then they feel light-headed and dizzy—and that's not good, either. You don't need to gulp air. Just breathe easily, the way you would if you were having a conversation.

Count Out Loud While You Exercise

There are two reasons to count out loud. First, it assures proper breathing— you can't hold your breath if you're speaking, and you're not likely to hyperventilate, either. Second, counting paces your lift and helps you move slowly. As you'll see in Chapter 8, we use the slow count of "1-2-3-Up; Pause; 1-2-3-Down."

Progress at the Recommended Pace

Some women become so enthusiastic about strength training that they press forward too quickly. As I'll explain in Chapter 9, you should select a weight for each exercise that you can lift in good form eight times in a row before your muscle becomes fatigued and needs to rest. If you use weights that are too heavy, you'll find it hard to maintain proper form, and you could hurt

CAUTION

I f you follow the instructions in this book, it's extremely unlikely that you'll ever experience any of the symptoms below. But if you do, use common sense: **Stop training immediately.** And if the symptom persists, contact your medical caregiver.

- ◆ Chest pain or pressure
- ◆ Dizziness or light-headedness
- ◆ Nausea
- ◆ Sweating not explained by physical effort or by hot flashes
- ◆ Any unusual or worsening pain—for instance, pain in a joint; or pain in the jaw or in the arm or shoulder that's not caused by muscle fatigue
- ◆ Flashes of light or other disturbances in vision

yourself. Also, your tendons and ligaments, which generally aren't as strong as your muscles, need time to catch up. When you progress slowly, everything gets strong together.

Do the exercises twice—or at most, three times—a week, with at least one day of rest in between. This level of challenge safely strengthens your muscles.

LISTEN TO YOUR BODY

I 'll tell you how much weight to lift during your first session, based on your answers to questions in Chapter 9. But after that, you're the one to decide if you stick with the same weight or increase it. So you'll need to understand your body's signals.

This program makes you stronger because it pushes your muscles to work near their capacity. If you select appropriate weights, your muscles will be tired as you complete the last few lifts of each exercise. The sensation should come on gradually and feel like the aching you experience anytime your muscles become fatigued. Once you stop, this mild discomfort should ease almost immediately. Sharp pain is another story, since it could indicate a mechanical problem or inflammation in a joint. (I'll provide more information about discomfort in Chapter 10.)

EIGHT EXERCISES
THAT WILL MAKE
YOU STRONG

This chapter tells you how to do the eight basic exercises of the *Strong Women Stay Young* Program. First you'll learn the moves. Then, in the next chapter, I'll explain how to customize the program so it's appropriate for you.

You'll start with relatively light weights—one to three pounds for each arm and three to five pounds for each leg, depending on your current strength. In the beginning you'll add weight every week. Within a few weeks you'll be training at the proper intensity: You'll be able to lift each weight eight times in good form, but this effort should be close to your limit. When the eighth lift is no longer a challenge, it's time to increase the load.

The program calls for two thirty-minute workouts per week. You'll do eight exercises that strengthen the major muscle groups of your legs and arms. As you read the descriptions, refer to the drawing on page 25, which shows these muscles. At the end of this chapter is a double-page chart illustrating all eight exercises—the *Strong Women Stay Young* Program at a glance.

ORDER OF EXERCISES

I've planned the order of the exercises to make your workouts efficient and comfortable. The first move, a chair stand, serves as a warm-up—it's important to warm your muscles to get them ready for exercise. The next three exercises focus on the large muscles of your lower body and are performed with ankle weights. Your whole body will warm up further as you do them. Two of these exercises require that you stand on one foot at a time, which can be tiring for the supporting leg. So there's a seated exercise in between.

When you finish the leg exercises, you can remove the ankle weights—this minimizes the time that the cuffs restrict your movement. Next you work your upper body with three dumbbell exercises. The last exercise, a toe stand, addresses balance as well as strength. As I'll explain in Chapter 10, it's not essential to do the exercises in this order. But I suggest you wait until you're familiar with the program to experiment.

LIFTS, REPS, AND SETS

In strength training, each complete move is called a **lift**. A series of lifts is referred to as **repetitions** or **reps**. In this program, eight reps make a **set**. You'll do two sets—a total of sixteen reps—for each exercise.

Each lift takes nine seconds: four seconds to raise the weight; a one-second pause for a breath; and four seconds to lower the weight. You'll stop for two or three seconds to take a breath between lifts. Since you'll use weights that you can't easily lift more than eight times, you'll need a longer rest—about a minute—between sets. It's not necessary to stop between exercises because different moves work different muscles, but you can rest for a minute or two if you wish.

RELAX!

In the instructions for each exercise, I'll remind you to check your body for tension—and to relax.

- **Face:** Don't furrow or knit your brow; keep your face relaxed.
- **Jaw and neck:** Avoid clenching your teeth or tightening your jaw. If your jaw is relaxed, your neck will be relaxed too.
- **Shoulders:** Don't scrunch your shoulders up toward your ears. Keep them back and relaxed.
- **Legs and arms:** Only the muscles you're exercising should be tensed. All other muscles in your body should be relaxed.

CHAIR STAND (WITHOUT WEIGHTS)

This super exercise tackles several important muscle groups at once. You'll strengthen and tone your thighs and work your back and abdominal muscles as well as your buttocks. Chair stands also improve your balance. Plus, this exercise is a great warm-up—which is why it comes first.

Starting position:

Sit toward the front of the chair seat, with your feet flat on the floor, shoulder-width apart. Cross your arms, and hold them against your chest, your left fingertips touching your right shoulder and your right fingertips touching your left shoulder.

▼ ▼ ▼ ▼ ▼ ▼ ▼ ▼ ▼ ▼ ▼ ▼ ▼ ▼ ▼ ▼ ▼ ▼ ▼

The move:

- **1-2-3-Up:** Keeping your back straight, lean forward slightly and stand up *slowly*. The entire effort should come from your leg and buttock muscles.
- **Pause** for a breath.
- **1-2-3-Down:** *Slowly* return to the starting position. Do not let yourself fall into the chair!
- **Pause** for a breath, then repeat.

Where you will feel the effort:

In your thighs and buttocks.

Reps and sets:

Do eight repetitions for one set. Rest for a minute, and do a second set.

Checklist:

The key to success with this exercise is to move slowly, especially as you return to the chair. Use your leg and buttock muscles to lower yourself—*don't* fall back into the seat. If the move is difficult, use your hands to make it easier. In a few weeks you should be able to do it without hands.

◆ Remember to move slowly.
◆ Lean just slightly forward as you start the move.
◆ Don't allow your knees to come in front of your toes.
◆ Don't hold your breath.
◆ Check for tension, and relax.

Put on your ankle weights for Exercises 2, 3, and 4.

Standing Leg Curl (with ankle weights)

The muscles along the backs of your thighs, just below your buttocks, are called the hamstrings. Any activity that uses your legs—walking, running, skiing, biking—will be more enjoyable as these muscles get stronger.

Starting position:

Stand just behind the chair, lightly holding the back for support. Your knees should just touch, and the fronts of your thighs should be even. Shift your body weight so that you are standing on your left leg.

The move:

- **1-2-3-Up:** Lift your right foot up until your thigh and lower leg form a ninety-degree angle. Your toes should point straight down at the top of the move.
- **Pause** for a breath.
- **1-2-3-Down:** Slowly lower your right foot until only the toes of that foot are in contact with the floor. Slide the toes of your right foot forward to the starting position.
- **Pause** for a breath. Then do the same move with your left leg. You will need to shift your weight from side to side as you change legs, but your torso should remain upright.

Where you will feel the effort:

On the back of the thigh you're lifting and also on the upper thigh of the supporting leg.

Reps and sets:

Repeat, alternating right and left legs until you have done eight leg curls with each leg—this is one set. Rest for a minute, and do a second set.

Checklist:

- Posture: Don't arch your back as you do the exercise.
- Your thighs should remain even and your knees touching throughout the move.

▼　▼　▼　▼　▼　▼　▼　▼　▼　▼　▼　▼　▼　▼　▼　▼　▼

- Don't let your knee or thigh move forward as the lower leg curls up.
- Don't hold your breath.
- Check for tension—and relax.

Knee Extension (with ankle weights)

This exercise strengthens the quadriceps, the large muscles in front
of your thighs. As your quads get stronger, your legs will become
shapelier—something you'll appreciate if you enjoy wearing shorts
or short skirts. And you'll notice a power difference when you walk,
climb stairs, bike, or engage in any sport that uses your legs.

Starting position:

Sit back in the chair. Your feet should be shoulder-width apart, with
your knees directly above them—your knees shouldn't touch each
other. Put the towel under your knees to pad them. Your toes should
just brush against the floor; if necessary, raise your knees by doubling

▼ ▼ ▼ ▼ ▼ ▼ ▼ ▼ ▼ ▼ ▼ ▼ ▼ ▼ ▼ ▼ ▼

up or rolling the towel. Rest your hands on top of your thighs or let them dangle at your sides; or lightly hold the edge of the chair seat.

The move:

- 1-2-3-Up: Slowly raise your right leg until the knee is as straight as possible. Keep your toes gently flexed up toward your body.
- **Pause** for a breath.
- 1-2-3-Down: Relax your ankle so your toes are no longer flexed up. Slowly lower your leg to the starting position.
- **Pause** for a breath. Then repeat the move with your left foot.

Where you will feel the effort:

On top of your upper thighs, with a stretching feeling in the backs of your thighs.

Reps and sets:

Repeat, alternating right and left legs until you have done eight knee extensions with each leg—this is one set. Rest for a minute, and do a second set.

Checklist:

- Posture: Don't arch your back as you do the exercise.
- Straighten your leg as far as possible at the end of the lift—the last part of the muscle contraction is the most important.
- Don't hold your breath.
- Check for tension—and relax.

SIDE HIP RAISE (WITH ANKLE WEIGHTS)

The hip abductors, the muscles that run along the outside of your thighs, help you maintain good balance—especially when you're making a side move. This exercise tones these muscles. You'll feel a difference when you dance, play tennis, or go skiing.

Starting position:

Stand behind the chair, holding the back lightly for support. Shift your body weight so that you are supported by your left leg. Your left knee should be straight (or very slightly bent) but not locked. Lift the right toes slightly. Be sure that your right foot points forward.

The move:

- ◆ **1-2-3-Up:** Slowly lift your leg out to the side until your foot is five to eight inches off the ground.
- ◆ **Pause** for a breath.
- ◆ **1-2-3-Down:** Slowly lower your leg to the starting position.
- ◆ **Pause** for a breath, then do the same move with your other leg. You will need to shift your weight from side to side as you change legs, but your torso should remain upright.

Where you will feel the effort:

On the outside of the thigh and buttock of the leg you're lifting, and also on the upper thigh of the nonlifting leg.

Reps and sets:

Repeat, alternating right and left legs, until you've completed eight side hip raises with each leg—one set. Rest for a minute, then do a second set.

Checklist:

- Your torso should remain upright during this exercise, not leaning to one side. If possible, check in a mirror to make sure your upper body isn't tilting.
- Keep your toes pointed forward throughout the move. Don't rotate your hip.
- Don't expect your foot to rise more than six to twelve inches off the floor. It's more beneficial to do the exercise in good form—with toes pointed straight forward, without rotating your hip, and not leaning your torso to the opposite side—than to lift your leg higher.
- Keep your fingertips on top of the chair for balance, but try not to grasp the chair tightly.
- Don't hold your breath.
- Check for tension—and relax.

When you've completed this exercise, take off your leg weights and put them in their container.

Biceps Curl (with dumbbells)

The biceps—the muscles in the front of your arm—are among the hardest-working muscles in your body. As they get stronger, everything you pick up seems to get lighter, whether it's groceries, toddlers, or suitcases packed for Tahiti. And if your lifestyle includes snow shoveling or rope climbing, this exercise will boost your performance. Don't worry about developing bulging Ms. Olympia biceps. This exercise firms and tones, so your arms will look shapely, not formidable.

Starting position:

Stand with your feet shoulder-width apart, with your arms down at your sides holding the dumbbells. Palms should face in, toward your legs.

The move:

◆ **1-2-3-Up:** Keeping your elbows gently pressed against your sides, raise the dumbbells by bringing your forearms up. The dumbbells should move from your sides to the front of your shoulders in one smooth motion. Your elbows will bend; your forearms will rotate; and your wrists will remain straight. At the end of the move, the dumbbells will be at shoulder height, parallel to the floor, with your palms facing your shoulders.

◆ **Pause** for a breath.

◆ **1-2-3-Down:** Lower your arms, smoothly rotating your forearms so the dumbbells return to the starting position, with palms facing in. Keep your elbows gently anchored at your sides through the entire movement.

◆ **Pause** for a breath, then repeat.

Where you will feel the effort:

In your upper arms.

Reps and sets:

Do eight repetitions for one set. Rest for a minute, and do a second set.

Checklist:

◆ Maintain good posture; don't arch your back.

◆ Don't bend your wrists.

◆ Keep your elbows anchored at your sides.

◆ Move slowly.

◆ Don't hold your breath.

◆ Check for tension—and relax.

Overhead Press (with dumbbells)

The triceps—the muscles in back of your upper arm—are notoriously weak. When you strengthen them with this exercise, you'll find it easier to tackle overhead tasks, such as changing ceiling lightbulbs or hoisting a heavy garment bag into the overhead compartment of an airplane. What's more, your upper arms will be tighter and trimmer. This move also works the deltoid and trapezius muscles of the upper back. So it's great for posture too.

Starting position:

Stand straight with a dumbbell in each hand. Hold the dumbbells up and parallel to the floor on either side of your shoulders. Your palms should be facing forward and there should be a straight line from the left dumbbell across your shoulders to the end of the right dumbbell.

The move:

- **1-2-3-Up:** Slowly push the dumbbells straight up over your head, keeping them in line with your body.
- **Pause** for a breath.
- **1-2-3-Down:** Return your arms to the starting position.
- **Pause** for a breath. Then repeat.

Where you will feel the effort:

In your back, shoulders, and the backs of your arms.

Reps and sets:

Do eight repetitions for one set. Rest for a minute, and do a second set.

Checklist:

- ◆ Maintain good posture throughout the move. Don't scrunch your shoulders!
- ◆ Be careful not to arch your back and put pressure on your lower spine.
- ◆ Don't hold your breath.
- ◆ Check for tension—and relax.

UPWARD ROW (WITH DUMBBELLS)

This exercise strengthens the deltoid (shoulder muscle), trapezius (upper back muscle), and biceps. Toning these muscles does more than improve your appearance in a tank top. The shoulder joint is one of the most important—and vulnerable—in the body. Strong shoulder muscles help stabilize this joint, allowing you to lift and carry heavy objects.

Starting position:

Stand with a dumbbell in each hand. Move your hands so that the dumbbells rest on the fronts of your thighs, with your palms facing your thighs.

The move:

- **1-2-3-Up:** Slowly pull the dumbbells upward along your torso until they are just below your chin. Keep your hands in the same position during the move; your wrists will bend to the side so your knuckles remain pointing down. At the end of the lift, your elbows will be at shoulder height and pointing out to the side; your forearms and the weights will be parallel to the floor.
- **Pause** for a breath.
- **1-2-3-Down:** Slowly lower the dumbbells to the starting position.
- **Pause** for a breath, then repeat.

Where you will feel the effort:

In your forearms, biceps, and shoulders.

Reps and sets:

Perform eight upward rows—one set. Put the weights down, and rest for a minute. Then do a second set.

Checklist:

- Don't scrunch your shoulders! That's the most common problem with this exercise.
- Make sure that your elbows and wrists are not above shoulder level.
- Maintain good posture.
- Don't hold your breath.
- Check for tension—and relax.

TOE STAND (WITHOUT WEIGHTS)

This is a three-purpose exercise, with a bonus. It improves your balance, makes your ankles more flexible, and strengthens the gastrocnemius and soleus muscles in the backs of your lower legs. You'll feel the difference when you're on your feet all day, because you use these muscles whenever you're standing. And the bonus is trimmer, more defined calves.

Instead of dumbbells and ankle cuffs, this exercise uses your body weight. Start with Level 1. If your calf muscles are weak or inflexible, you may not be able to raise yourself very much. Work first on improving the strength of these muscles until you can lift yourself all the way up onto your toes. When Level 1 is no longer a challenge even without help from your hands, move to Level 2, which is performed on a step.

TOE STAND—LEVEL I

Starting position:

Stand twelve inches away from a wall, with your feet about twelve inches apart. Rest your fingertips lightly on the wall to help maintain your balance. As you improve, try to become less reliant on the wall. For safety's sake, always perform this exercise with a wall in front of you.

The move:

- **1-2-3-Up:** Slowly raise yourself as high as possible on the balls of both feet.
- **1-2-3-Hold:** Remain on your toes for another count of three, breathing normally.

- ◆ **1-2-3-Down:** Slowly lower yourself to the starting position.
- ◆ **Pause** for a breath and repeat.

Reps and sets:

Repeat eight times—one set. Rest for a minute, and do a second set.

TOE STAND—LEVEL 2

Starting position:

Stand on the bottom step of a staircase with a sturdy railing you can hold on to. Place the balls of your feet on the step, with your heels off the edge. Hold on to the railing, and slowly lower your heels as far as possible.

The move:

- **1-2-3-Up:** Slowly raise yourself as high as possible on the balls of both feet.
- **1-2-3-Hold:** Remain on your toes for another count of three, breathing normally.
- **1-2-3-Down:** Slowly lower yourself to the starting position.
- **Pause** for a breath and repeat.

Reps and sets:

Repeat eight times—one set. Rest for a minute, then do a second set.

TOE STAND—FOR BOTH LEVELS

Where you will feel the effort:

In your ankles, feet, and the backs of your calves.

Checklist:

- Maintain good upright posture.
- Do the toe stands slowly—many people have a tendency to raise and lower themselves too quickly. In fact, you'll benefit even more if you maintain the position for fifteen to thirty seconds rather than just three seconds.
- Don't hold your breath.
- Check for tension—and relax.

COOL-DOWN

I recommend that you cool down with a stretch after a strength-training session. This will enhance improvements in flexibility and relieve any tightness you might feel.

Select three or more of the exercises that are performed with weights—as many as you wish. Do each move two or three times *without* weights, going through the full range of motion very slowly. Hold the fully extended position for fifteen to thirty seconds each time—*and never bounce.*

For more suggestions, read the classic book on the subject: *Stretching,* by Bob Anderson (Shelter Publications, 1987).

STRONG WOMEN
STAY YOUNG

#1: CHAIR STAND

#2: STANDING LEG CURL

#3: KNEE EXTENSION

#4: SIDE HIP RAISE

Eight Exercises That Will Make You Strong

#5: BICEPS CURL

#6: OVERHEAD PRESS

#7: UPWARD ROW

#8: TOE STAND

LEVEL 1

LEVEL 2

CREATING AN INDIVIDUALIZED PROGRAM

Y ou've learned how to do the moves. The next step is to turn the exercises into an *individualized program* that will increase your strength. This program will be simple—but not easy. To get strong, you must train at a challenging level. And as you become stronger, you'll need to adjust to maintain that challenge. Using the right weights for each exercise is the key to both safety and success. If you overdo, you'll find the program unnecessarily difficult. On the other hand, if you expect too little of yourself, you won't progress.

WHERE TO START

T he greatest amount of weight you can lift just once is your maximum strength capacity. In this program, you'll be working out at 70 to 80 percent of your maximum. This is high enough to push your muscles to become stronger, yet well within your ability. For the sake of safety, though, you'll start at a level that's considerably lower—about 50 to 60 percent. This gives you time to learn the moves and minimizes the risk of injury if you make errors in form at the beginning.

Since you use your muscles in everyday life, it's easy to approximate your current strength. The simple test below lets you determine a safe starting point for the program. If you're unsure how to answer, err on the side of underestimating rather than overestimating your strength.

Directions: For each of these three activities, check the column that best describes how strong you are.

	A	B	C
Walking and running			
I can run a mile without resting. (Check column A)			
I can walk a mile without resting, but couldn't run. (Check column B)			
I can't walk a mile without resting. (Check column C)			
Climbing stairs			
I can climb five flights of stairs without a pause. (Check column A)			
I can climb two to four flights without a pause. (Check column B)			
I can't climb two flights of stairs without a pause. (Check column C)			

	A	B	C
Carrying heavy grocery bags* I can carry one bag in each arm. (Check column A) I can carry one bag with both arms. (Check column B) I can't carry such a bag for this distance. (Check column C) *Assume you're carrying fifteen-pound grocery bags into the house and that the bags are carried in your arms, not by handles.			
Number of checks in each column			

- If you had even one check in column C, start at the **beginning** level.
- If you had a combination of checks in columns A and B, start at the **intermediate** level.
- If you had three checks in column A, start at the **advanced** level.

STARTING LEVEL	POUNDS FOR EACH ARM	POUNDS FOR EACH LEG
Beginning	1	2
Intermediate	2	3
Advanced	3	4

Once you've established your starting level, use the table on the previous page to determine the number of pounds to use for your leg and arm weights during your first session.

Don't hesitate to start at a lower level if you're concerned that these weights might be too heavy. For instance, if you've had problems with a knee and want to make sure you don't strain it, begin with lighter leg weights— or even no weights—and increase cautiously.

Your first few sessions probably will seem easy, but in my experience that's helpful when you're learning the exercises and proper form. Within a

IF YOU HAVE A SPECIFIC HEALTH CONCERN

At Tufts, we've seen strength training benefit the frail elderly, people who have recovered from major surgery (including joint replacement, hysterectomy, mastectomy, and other cancer treatment), as well as individuals with chronic but stable medical conditions such as osteoporosis, heart disease, diabetes, rheumatoid arthritis, osteoarthritis, and other joint problems.

Here are general recommendations for those with medical problems:

- ♦ Be sure to discuss the program with your doctor before you start, so you can make any necessary adjustments.
- ♦ Start conservatively and progress slowly. For instance, your doctor may suggest that you begin the arm exercises without dumbbells. Then, if that's comfortable, you could try one-pound dumbbells and increase the weights every two weeks instead of weekly.
- ♦ Consider working with a personal trainer, at least for a few sessions, to make sure your form is correct.
- ♦ Pay attention to your body. Feeling good is the best indication that you're exercising properly.

few sessions you'll reach the right intensity. Thereafter you'll add weight as your muscles strengthen. **The program will always match your body.**

HOW TO EVALUATE
YOUR EFFORT

Many researchers use a twenty-point scale, called the Borg Exercise Intensity Scale, that helps participants translate into a single number what it feels like to make a certain physical effort. For this book, I've created a simpler five-point version. Though it's a subjective measurement, this scale will help you recognize when you're working out at the right intensity.

The right effort for strength training is Level 4. You should find the weight moderately difficult to lift the first time but well within your capability. By the third or fourth lift, it should seem heavier. Ideally, you should be able to perform the eighth lift in good form, but feel that if you didn't stop and rest your muscles, you couldn't continue.

Working out at Level 3 (except for the first few weeks) is not sufficiently challenging; it will increase your endurance but not your strength. On the other hand, training at Level 5 is risky—if the effort is too great, you won't be able to maintain proper form—and you might injure yourself.

FINDING THE
RIGHT CHALLENGE

Because I've given you a very conservative starting point, the effort during your first two strength-training sessions will probably be at Level 3 or even Level 2. That's not a problem. Learning the exercises is sufficient challenge. Focus on your form, on breathing and relaxing, and on establishing the slow rhythm of lifting and lowering a weight. You may find it helpful to photocopy the chart on pages 144 to 145 for quick reference.

During the first week, stay at the starting level to learn the exercises, even if it's too easy. If your workout seems too hard, or if your muscles are very uncomfortable afterward, drop down a pound.

EXERCISE INTENSITY SCALE	
EXERCISE INTENSITY LEVEL	DESCRIPTION OF EFFORT
1	Very easy: Too easy to be noticed, like lifting a pencil.
2	Easy: Can be felt, but isn't fatiguing, like carrying a book.
3	Moderate: Fatiguing only if prolonged, like carrying a full handbag that seems heavier as the day goes on.
4	Hard: More than moderate at first, and becomes difficult by the time you complete six or seven repetitions. You can make the effort eight times in good form, but need to rest afterward.
5	Extremely hard: Requires all your strength, like lifting a piece of heavy furniture that you can raise only once, if at all.

In the second week, add up to one pound per session to your arm and leg weights, as needed to increase effort to Level 4. Don't add weight if your muscles are sore—continue with the same weight or decrease the weight if the discomfort is bothersome. By the end of the third or fourth week, you should be working out at Level 4 on all the exercises.

You may reach Level 4 sooner on some exercises than on others. If one of the arm exercises isn't challenging enough, use a heavier dumbbell for that lift, even if you aren't ready to increase weight for a different arm exercise. For instance, you'll probably need a heavier weight for the biceps curl than for the overhead press.

With the leg exercises, you're likely to find that the knee extensions are a little easier than the standing leg curl or side hip raise. Unfortunately, it's inconvenient to remove the ankle cuffs and change the weights. You may be able to make quick adjustments by slipping a one- or two-pound pellet under the belt that holds the ankle weight snug. That way you could increase the weight for the knee extension without taking off the cuffs.

RECORDING YOUR PROGRESS

If we were working together, we'd keep records of your progress, because nothing is more exciting and encouraging. I urge you to copy the form on the next page and fill it in after each workout. You're doing eight exercises twice a week, and you're changing one or more weights nearly every time you work out. So it's easy to forget which weight goes with which move. Your workouts will be faster if you don't have to stop to remember what you did the last time.

STRONG WOMEN STAY YOUNG
WEEKLY STRENGTH-TRAINING LOG

EXERCISES 2 SETS/8 REPS	DATE: POUNDS OR LEVEL	DATE: POUNDS OR LEVEL	COMMENTS
Chair stand			
Standing leg curl			
Knee extension			
Side hip raise			
Biceps curl			
Overhead press			
Upward row			
Toe stand			

WHAT TO EXPECT DURING THE FIRST THREE MONTHS

The first three months of a strength-training program are a very special time. You're forming a habit that can truly change the course of your life. During this period you can expect exciting improvements—this is the time when change is most rapid.

Month 1: You'll learn the exercises, using light weights initially. Your first sessions may take longer than an hour, but you'll soon become more efficient. Some women experience minor aches and pains during the first two weeks, especially if they aren't already fit. I'll have suggestions in Chapter 10 for dealing with this temporary discomfort. By the end of the first month the exercises will be familiar, and you'll be performing them at— or at least close to—the proper intensity.

Month 2: This is when women start to see payoffs. For some exercises you may be lifting *twice* as much weight as you did at the beginning. Many women notice that they feel stronger and more energetic. If you were sedentary before, you may notice changes in everyday activities. If you were already fit, improvements may be evident only when you push yourself—for instance, you may be less tired than usual after a run.

Month 3: You're entering a new and important phase of strength training—the time when your muscles themselves begin to change. Your initial gains came mostly from newly activated nerves, as I explained in Chapter 2. Change will become slower now. You'll add weight less often— maybe every two or three weeks—but a lot is happening! Your muscle cells are getting bigger, and your bones are starting their slow reaction to the stimulus of strength training.

Many women feel revitalized after three months on this program. They have more energy and move more quickly. Some lose weight; others slim down because once-flabby spots have firmed up. The weaker and more out-of-shape you were at the beginning, the more noticeable the improvements. Some of the most important changes are invisible, however. The fact that you're stronger means your muscles and bones have benefited. You can't actually see these changes without sophisticated tests, but you can be sure they've occurred.

WORKING TOWARD GOALS

After the first month, try to increase the weight for each exercise every week or two. I'm not suggesting that you overdo by attempting to work out at Level 5. But you'll make more progress if you push yourself to stay at the top of the Level 4 range rather than waiting until the effort drops to Level 3 before you increase the weight.

Weekly changes won't always be possible. You'll soon see that progress is made more easily on some exercises than on others. Moreover, if you buy five-, eight-, and ten-pound dumbbells—which is what I suggest to keep expenses in bounds—you'll make bigger but less frequent jumps with your arm weights. As an interim step you can do just the second set with the heavier weight. Then the next session, try to use the heavier weight for both sets.

I've observed many people as they follow this program, and I'm still struck by the wide range of individual responses. Some move forward rapidly; others advance more slowly. Progress can be uneven. One woman may quickly gain strength in her arms, while another sees the biggest change in her legs. There are certain common patterns, though: Most people find the biceps curl and the upward row are considerably easier than the overhead press. That's because the triceps is a much smaller muscle that gets less exercise in everyday life. Similarly, it's usual for the knee extension to be easier than the side hip raise and standing leg curl.

The following table shows strength goals by age and exercise. When you're training at these levels, you will have obtained most of the health benefits you can expect from a strengthening program—provided you keep it up. Most women reach these goals after six to nine months on this program, or at least come very close. And others go past them. As I mentioned in Chapter 2, researchers who've followed people for two years find they keep improving, albeit at a very slow rate.

How much further should you go? That's up to you. Some women are eager to press on. Here are my recommendations if you want to advance past the goals in this book:

◆ For your legs: Don't go above twenty pounds with the ankle weights—heavier versions may create orthopedic problems. Instead, switch to exercises that use your body weight for resistance, which you can find in many books. (See the list of books on page 203.) Another option that's practical for some women: Use strength-training machines.

◆ For your arms: Don't lift dumbbells that are heavier than twenty-five pounds—they're too unsteady. If you want to go past twenty-five pounds, use barbells, which are more stable. You can do the biceps curls, overhead press, and upward row with barbells. Or switch to machines for the arm exercises.

Please remember that after you've been strength training for six months, improvements will come more slowly. I think it's better to maintain these healthy levels than to struggle to surpass them—and risk becoming discouraged or bored. Greater benefits can be realized by adding new strengthening exercises, such as moves for the back and abdomen. Chapter 11 provides some suggestions.

STRENGTH-TRAINING GOALS
(POUNDS AND LEVELS)

EXERCISE	AGE 49 AND YOUNGER	AGE 50 TO 69	AGE 70 AND OLDER
Standing leg curl	10 to 14	8 to 12	6 to 10
Knee extension	15 to 20	12 to 18	10 to 15
Side hip raise	12 to 18	10 to 14	8 to 12
Biceps curl	12 to 20	10 to 15	8 to 12
Overhead press	12 to 18	8 to 12	6 to 10
Upward row	12 to 20	10 to 15	8 to 12
Toe stand	Level 2	Level 2	Level 2

STAYING ON TRACK

◆ ◆ ◆

I feel so much better, and I am amazed that I actually enjoy this stuff. I had spent my whole life believing I did not like exercise. Of course, I had never tried it. It's just so much easier to live when you feel healthy. Cleaning the house used to be a nightmare. Now I whiz through it on my way to something else. I do so much more—I even took up art classes and find time to paint as well.

    —Susan

Strength training is the perfect complement to running. I used to have a slight bit of knee pain after a run, but no longer. Hill running is easier too. I always felt terrific from running. But combined with the strength training, I have never felt better in my life—or looked better. People at work have noticed something different and ask me what the secret is.

    —Sherry

◆ ◆ ◆

'm very proud that nearly everyone who joined my *JAMA* study stayed to the end. The only exception was a woman who had to leave because of an unrelated health problem. All the other volunteers came faithfully, twice a week for a full year. Yes, they missed a session here and there—but only about one workout a month. This is one of the highest attendance rates ever achieved by an exercise study that lasted so long.

Obviously, I can't give you the individual attention these women received. But that was just one explanation for their perseverance. The main reason was **they felt so great about what was happening to their bodies, they didn't want to stop.** Flora was one of the volunteers in the strength-training group. She says:

> *You can't imagine how good you can feel until you do something like this. I still go twice a week. It would be silly not to.*

I wish I could wave a magic wand to make sure you'll remain as excited and enthusiastic as you are right now. Unfortunately, there is no magic. Only your own determination will keep you on track for the time it takes to make this program a permanent way of life. However, I *can* give you proven strategies. Use them—they really help.

MAKE A COMMITMENT TO FOLLOW THE PROGRAM FOR AT LEAST FOUR WEEKS

What's so special about four weeks? Two things:

- ♦ It takes about that long to settle into this program. You have to become familiar with the equipment, learn the exercises, find the right intensity, and set up a good routine.
- ♦ This is about the time when you start to see changes. Remember Jayne from Chapter 5, who had a hard time starting? After she'd been doing the program for about a month, she had a startling experience:

My fingers happened to brush against the back of my right thigh, and I felt a hard oval lump there. My heart started racing. I felt the back of my left thigh and found the same lump. You have to remember that I'd never exercised before. It took me quite a few minutes to realize that what I was feeling was muscles.

After four weeks, you're no longer a beginner. But you need at least eight more weeks (and often longer) for a change in behavior to become a habit—something that's part of your life and that you actually enjoy doing.

KEEP LOGS

Study after study has shown that if you record your progress in a fitness program, you're much more likely to be successful. I strongly encourage you to copy the form on page 153 and keep logs—at least through the first twelve weeks.

Record-keeping helps in two ways:

- ◆ **Motivation:** These exercises improve your strength and health relatively quickly, but it doesn't happen overnight. A log helps you see progress achieved over weeks and months—and that encourages you to accomplish even more.
- ◆ **Efficiency:** Workouts go more quickly and smoothly when you keep records. Charlotte comments:

If I didn't write down what weights I lifted, the logic in the program would be shot. I'd do ten pounds one week, two the next. So it's essential for me to keep a record. I don't even wait for the session to be over; I write down the weight right after I do the exercise—it's become a habit. I have a lot of data, and it's very nice to see.

So take the time—just a few seconds, really—to fill out the logs. **This is probably the single most important step you can take to assure your success.**

ENJOY YOUR WORKOUTS

M any women take pleasure from the pure physical sensation of lifting weights. Ursula is one of them:

> *I like the pulling of the weight and the stretching out. I feel I'm taking time for myself. I put on music; I move slowly and rhythmically. I find it has a contemplative quality. Afterward I'm very refreshed.*

You might find the moves intriguing for the first month or so, then get restless when the novelty wears off. Don't stop! There are many ways to boost your enjoyment:

Find a Workout Style That Motivates You

Sarah and Ursula were part of a small group that met weekly to test the exercises in the first edition of this book. Each followed the program in her own style.

Sarah wanted to see results:

> *In the first two months, I made a lot of progress on two of the arm exercises—biceps curl and upward row—but the triceps exercise was stuck at five pounds. I found that demoralizing. My next dumbbell was eight pounds, but one day I decided what the heck. And guess what: I could do it. That gave me such a boost that I began pushing myself a little harder.*

Ursula took a very different approach:

> *There are so many things I've got to confront myself with, and I didn't want this to become a source of stress. I progress more slowly than anyone else in the group. But instead of thinking at*

the end of the set, "Good, this is going to be the last lift," I actually enjoy it.

I think they're both right! The important thing is to do this program the way that makes you enjoy it and stick with it. And as long as you progress, no matter how slowly, you'll realize the benefits.

Devise Positive Distractions

Some women laughingly admit that strength training gives them an excuse to watch TV "trash" they secretly enjoy. Others listen to music or recorded books. Andrea, a reader from Australia, wrote:

One of the attractions of this program to me is that I can incorporate it into my time at home while watching TV or listening to the radio or—when I feel really hyped—to very loud CDs (although having one's feet glued to the floor by twenty kilos of weights makes bopping a bit limited).

Work Out with a Friend or Form a Group

Having an exercise partner is the next best thing to hiring a professional trainer. It gives you the structure of a regular schedule and a commitment to someone else. You and your partner can check each other's form—this is especially handy in the beginning. And of course, your workouts will be more fun. If one of you hits a low point, the other can provide a boost. Daughters and mothers make excellent exercise partners.

Here at Tufts, colleagues commonly exercise together before work or during lunch hour. You might be able to recruit neighbors or members of a community organization. Strength training is an ideal exercise for a group. Because you're standing or sitting in one place, it's easy to socialize. And since everyone does the same moves, even if they're lifting different weights, your partners don't need to be evenly matched as they would for tennis or walking.

Two readers who live in the same condo building—Mary Lou and Sara—have been strength training together for more than a year. They keep their weights in Mary Lou's apartment, and twice a week Sara comes over for a workout. Says Mary Lou:

We talk, laugh, take turns counting while the other gabs. One day Sara called to say she had to wait for repairmen to finish a job, so we would have to cancel our session. I told her I had an idea and would be at her door in a few minutes. She said "But what about all the weights?" I told her not to worry. In a few minutes, I knocked on her door and said, "Good afternoon, ma'am, welcome to Weights on Wheels." I had gone down to the basement and brought up one of the carts the building keeps in the basement to bring up groceries. So we had our workout and a good laugh!

Swap Exercises

Another way to make sessions more enjoyable—especially after you've been doing the program for several months—is to make a few changes in the exercises. See Chapter 11 for options.

Change Your Schedule

Some people prefer shorter and more frequent sessions. That's perfectly okay. For instance, you could do the arm exercises one day and leg exercises the next. Here are some points to remember:

- ◆ Allow the muscles you're training to rest for a day between workouts.
- ◆ Warm your muscles before you lift weights. You can use

the chair stands as a warm-up. (Yes, that exercise can be repeated without a day of rest in between.) Five minutes of aerobic activity—brisk walking, marching in place, climbing stairs—also serves as a warm-up.
◆ Include a cool-down and stretch in each workout session. (See page 143.)

KEEP COMFORTABLE

Pain or injury can derail an exercise program. Fortunately, these problems are not common with strength training. Here's what you need to know to minimize discomfort:

◆ ANTICIPATE A LITTLE MUSCLE SORENESS AT FIRST

Your body isn't accustomed to lifting heavy weights. Also, this program works your muscles through a larger range of motion than they're used to. So it's not surprising that you may feel mild achiness during the first few weeks of the program or after you return to it following a lengthy absence. (Also, some people run into problems because they get too enthusiastic and push themselves too hard.)

In the first week, you may feel fine during the session itself, then develop aches the next day. This is the **delayed muscle soreness** I mentioned in Chapter 2. It's caused by eccentric muscle contractions—the part of the lift when you lower the weight. Particular muscles may feel sore, or you might experience a general achiness as if you were coming down with the flu.

Whatever the cause, muscle soreness is usually mild and gone within two days. I don't recommend a painkiller—not even aspirin or another over-the-counter drug like ibuprofen. Medication may interfere with the body's natural repair process, which is what helps build muscles. For relief, try these measures instead:

◆ Gently stretch your muscles by performing the exercises very slowly and smoothly, without weights.

- ♦ Soak in a hot bath to relax.
- ♦ Massage the muscle (if you can reach it). If you really want to pamper yourself, have a professional massage.

♦ LEARN THE DIFFERENCE BETWEEN "GOOD" AND "BAD" PAIN

After the first few sessions, you're much less likely to experience pain. But if you do, you need to understand it. Pain comes in different forms and means different things.

"Good" pain isn't a sign of trouble; it's muscle fatigue. Your muscles *should* feel fatigued by the end of eight repetitions in a high-intensity strength-training program like this one. What you're feeling is burning from lactic acid—a muscle's normal response to hard work. The burn should disappear in minutes as the lactic acid is broken down by your body. Here's how Sarah describes the sensations:

> *My muscles hurt more and more in the second half of the second set. For instance, when I'm doing the biceps curl, my arm feels the way it did when I was in school and carried heavy books around all day. When I'm done—finally!—the pain goes away nearly instantly and is replaced by a warm glowing feeling in the muscle. This is actually very pleasant.*

The exercises should never be sharply painful—if they are, that's "bad" pain, and it's a signal to stop. Sharp pain doesn't necessarily mean you've injured yourself by lifting weights; more likely, a preexisting joint problem has become evident because the joint is being worked instead of pampered.

How can you tell the good pain from the bad when you're strength-training? Here's a guide to the key differences:

	GOOD PAIN	**BAD PAIN**
Sensation	Dull ache	Sharp pain
Location	In the muscle	In or near the joint
After exercise	Relieved within minutes	Continues to hurt
Next session	Same effort is less painful	No improvement or worse
What it means	Normal muscle fatigue	Problem with a joint or muscle

Here are some guidelines for responding to bad pain:

♦ Stop the exercise. The pain will probably go away by itself. If not, you can speed it along by elevating the joint and icing it. If the pain is severe and gets worse, seek medical attention.

♦ During the next exercise session try again, but cautiously. Use lighter weights and a more limited range of motion. If that goes well for two sessions, slowly increase the weights and range of motion.

♦ Don't take painkillers unless your doctor advises it. Medicine can mask the pain—which is a warning from your body—and mislead you into thinking you can exercise when you really shouldn't.

♦ If the pain persists for two or more sessions, seek medical attention.

HELP! I'VE GONE OFF TRACK!

Sometimes a woman starts the program with great enthusiasm—then finds she's not doing it the way she had intended. She feels guilty and resolves to try harder. But that doesn't help either.

If this happens to you, don't despair: *It's never too late to get going again.*

◆ "I Never Really Started"

Don't give up! Set an easier short-term goal, to give yourself the satisfaction of success. Instead of trying to do the program twice a week, pick a time and aim to do it just once a week for the next three weeks. That's only three sessions, which may not sound like much. But achieving a goal can really turn things around. When you've established a routine for one session per week, consider adding the second session. If all you can manage is one weekly workout, continue with that. You'll benefit, though your progress will be slower.

◆ "I Can't Seem to Do It Twice a Week"

Some women never plan their workouts, and they do just fine. It's never the same time from one session to the next, but twice a week they manage to find a spare thirty minutes and they lift weights.

If spontaneity works for you, that's great. But many of us require more structure. If you find you're missing the second session nearly every week, take that as a signal that you need to set aside regular times for your workouts.

If you don't seem to have a minute to spare, take another look at Chapter 5, where I have many practical suggestions for busy women.

◆ "I'm Going Out of Town—What Should I Do?"

Even if you can't take your weights along, you don't have to abandon your program. Here are some possibilities:

- Stay at a hotel that has a fitness center, as many now do.
- Do strengthening exercises that require only your body weight (see page 205).
- Be as active as you can while you're away. That's easy if you're sightseeing. But even if you're on a business trip, look for opportunities to give yourself a mini-workout: Walk when possible; take the stairs instead of the elevator; carry your own luggage.
- Most important of all: **When you return, resume your program right away.** It's so easy to give yourself a few extra days off—and let them stretch into weeks or even months. Don't worry if you need to drop back a little, because you'll soon catch up.

MAINTAINING YOUR SUCCESS

After twelve weeks on this program, you will have made significant gains in strength. Sometime in the six months after that, improvements usually slow down. At that point, you'll probably be lifting weights within the ranges I suggested as goals in Chapter 9. Continuing at this level will preserve everything you've gained. You can try to increase further, but you won't win additional health benefits if you do. It's much better, I think, to enjoy your workouts at the target level than to push yourself and risk turning the program into an unpleasant chore.

Dealing with Temporary Setbacks

By now the program will have become a normal part of your life, something you do automatically. Indeed, you may find that if you miss a few sessions, your body actually craves the exercises.

Nobody is perfect, however. It's not realistic to expect that you'll always do the program twice a week, fifty-two weeks a year. Disruptions are part of life. You might get married, have a baby, move, change jobs, start school, get sick. When you're in the midst of a major upheaval, anything less urgent is set aside—and that's understandable. Allow yourself to deal with these events, even if that means being less consistent about strength training.

I hope you won't panic or feel guilty if you miss a few weeks when life becomes complicated. But it's important to limit this period and to return to the program when you can. If you do, the setback will be temporary.

You might also consider what an exercise program can do for you during a period of adversity. One woman in my study, who was coping with a serious illness in her family, told me:

> Working out relieves stress. I leave everything at the doorstep when I come to the gym. Afterward I definitely feel better. I have a new outlook.

If you can't get back into the groove, reread Chapter 5—all the suggestions for starting apply to restarting as well.

Adding Aerobic Exercise

Strength training has many benefits for health and well-being, but it doesn't train your heart and lungs. For that essential piece of the fitness picture, you need aerobic activity. An aerobic activity is any exercise that speeds up your heartbeat and your breathing rate. Examples are brisk walking, running, rowing, stair climbing, and even house cleaning at a rapid pace.

Aerobic exercise helps you live better as well as longer. Consider this dazzling list of benefits—all of which come without worrisome side effects:

- ◆ Improves the health of the lungs and cardiovascular system
- ◆ Helps tone muscles
- ◆ Contributes to weight loss: consumes calories; helps burn fat in the abdominal area; tames the appetite
- ◆ Provides emotional benefits: boosts self-esteem; safely relieves depression, anxiety, stress, and insomnia

The best news of all is that it doesn't take a lot to make a major difference. If you compare the health of very sedentary people—their cardiovascular fitness, their incidence of diseases like diabetes, their longevity, and so on—to that of professional athletes, the jocks are way ahead. No surprise there. But what's interesting is that if you look at people along the whole spectrum, the fitness graph isn't a straight line. It turns out that the biggest jump comes at the very bottom of the range, when our couch potato clicks off the remote and stands up.

In other words, the less active you are now, the more benefit you get from adding even a small amount of exercise to your life.

The research evidence is so overwhelming that the 1996 Surgeon General's Report on Physical Activity and Health declared that **moderate exercise is just as essential to a healthy life as good nutrition, seat belts, and avoiding cigarettes.** How much is enough? Just thirty minutes a day suffices.

You may already meet this standard. If not—and unfortunately, this is the case with most women—I hope you'll make the federal guidelines into a personal goal. When people tell me they have no time, I always ask them, *"Do you want to take time when you're in your fifties, sixties, seventies to care for your diabetes? Or to be in the hospital with heart disease and bone fractures?"*

No matter how busy you are, you can find thirty minutes. It doesn't have to be a solid block of time—three ten-minute snatches will do the trick. And "moderate exercise" doesn't necessarily mean sports or something you do at the gym while wearing a jogging suit. Any activity that raises your heart rate and body temperature counts. If you take a ten-minute walk to the bus in the morning, run around the yard with your kids for ten minutes in the afternoon, and spend another ten minutes in the evening doing a quick cleanup with the vacuum, that does it!

Unfortunate, but true: The more unfit you are, and the more you need to be active, the less fun it is to exercise. Who wants to take a walk if your legs ache and you become winded after five minutes? This is where strength training makes a great difference. Becoming stronger can turn around the negative cycle in which inactivity leads to weakness, which makes movement harder, which leads to further inactivity. Instead, by becoming stronger, you can do more and more—and I hope you will.

MY SIMPLE PERSONAL PLAN FOR STAYING ACTIVE

exercise regularly, but I also make a point of tucking a little extra activity into my life. Here's how:

♦ **I use myself for transportation**

Several days a week, I take a train from my home to a station in downtown Boston that's a little over a mile from my office. From there I can take the subway—or I can walk. The walk takes me twenty-two minutes. On average, the subway takes a total of fifteen minutes. So my twenty-two-minute walk "costs" just seven minutes of extra time.

Over the weekend, I look for opportunities to walk or ride my bike. On family excursions to the center of town, which is a mile and a half away, I drive the kids in one direction while my husband walks or bikes; going home, we swap. This way each of us gets an exercise break without imposing on the other.

♦ **I take the stairs instead of the elevator**

I work in a high-rise building, on the fourteenth floor, and I make a point of going up the stairs whenever possible. The climb takes five minutes. Many people are astonished when I tell them this—yet they wouldn't be at all surprised if I said that I work out on a stair climber for five minutes.

♦ **I use phone time for an exercise break**

During long calls at work, I reach under my desk and grab the ten-pound dumbbell I keep there for just these occasions. While I talk, my biceps and triceps get a workout. Or I do the toe stands.

♦ **I select physically demanding leisure activities**

Among my favorites are cross-country skiing, hiking, biking, running, and swimming.

FOR FURTHER INFORMATION ON FITNESS AND AEROBIC EXERCISE

Shape Up America!, a program launched by Dr. C. Everett Koop to promote physical fitness, has superb booklets on nutrition and exercise—and they're free! To request *Fitting Fitness In*, which offers ninety-nine practical tips, write to: Shape Up America, 6707 Democracy Boulevard, Suite 306, Bethesda, MD 20817. The Shape Up America Web site (http://www.shapeup.org/sua) provides self-tests and helpful fitness information, or call 301-493-5368.

Another excellent online resource is Fitness Link (http://www.fitnesslink.com). The site contains exercise information and extensive lists of links on fitness.

If you want to become more active, these three books are excellent guides:

- *Biomarkers: The 10 Determinants of Aging You Can Control*, by William Evans, Ph.D., and Irwin H. Rosenberg, M.D., with Jacqueline Thompson (Simon & Schuster, 1992).
- *The Wellness Guide to Lifelong Fitness*, by Timothy P. White, Ph.D., and the editors of the University of California at Berkeley Wellness Letter (REBUS, distributed by Random House, 1993).
- *Fitness and Health*, by Brian Sharkey, Ph.D. (Human Kinetics, 1996).

IV

A LIFETIME OF FITNESS

▼ ▼ ▼ ▼

MORE

STRENGTHENING

EXERCISES

Once your arms and legs are stronger, I hope you'll go beyond the eight exercises of the *Strong Women Stay Young* Program. In Chapter 10, I offered suggestions for becoming more active. This chapter provides additional strength-training exercises that can supplement your basic workout. The new moves target important muscle groups—in the upper and lower back, the abdomen, and the shoulders—that are often weak in women.

Valuable as they are, I didn't include these exercises in the basic program because most are performed on the floor. Many women tell me it's hard for them to get down on the floor—and even worse, get up again! I didn't want that problem to discourage anyone from trying this program. If you felt the same way before you started, I hope you'll have a change of heart now that you're stronger.

Here's what the new exercises can do for you:

♦ FIRM AND FLATTEN YOUR ABDOMEN

"What can I do to trim my tummy?" I hear this question every time I speak to a community group, whether the audience is teenagers, new moms, or senior citizens. Their motive may be appearance, but important health issues are at stake too. That stubborn midsection bulge involves body fat as well as flabby muscles—and excess abdominal fat is associated with greater health risks for women than excess fat in the thighs and buttocks. The solution requires a combination of strength training to tone the abdominal muscles (see page 178), plus aerobic exercise and (usually) weight loss to reduce fat.

♦ STRENGTHEN YOUR SHOULDERS AND BACK

Many women suffer from shoulder or back pain. Shoulders are the trickiest joint in the body because they move in many directions. Strength training makes shoulders stronger and increases their range of motion, which reduces the risk of injury.

Jill, whose family history of osteoporosis was mentioned in Chapter 3, also has a heritage of back problems:

> My grandmother called her spasms "Hexenschussen"; my mother said her "sacroiliac went out"; and I'm just stuck with lower-back problems. Imagine my surprise when the very weakness I feared might worsen with exercise cleared up totally once my abs got into shape.

♦ RESHAPE YOUR BODY

Strength training doesn't perform plastic surgery, but you'd be surprised at what it can accomplish by trimming fat and defining your muscles. You can make a flat, droopy bottom firmer and rounder; you can tighten those "wings" under your upper arms.

CAUTION

If you have a back problem or have had one in the past, please check with your medical practitioner before adding the back or abdominal exercises. You may be steered to other exercises that are more appropriate for your condition.

◆ REFRESH YOUR WORKOUTS AND EXPAND YOUR REPERTOIRE

Adding new exercises is a great way to keep from getting stale. Also, new moves allow you to adapt to new circumstances. For instance, most of the exercises in this chapter use your body weight, not equipment, for resistance. This makes it easier to keep up with your program when you're away from home.

When should you add new exercises? I suggest you wait until you've mastered the basic eight exercises and established a regular weekly routine for strength training. That usually takes about three months. At that point you can decide what you'd like to try next. I'll have some suggestions at the end of the chapter for developing new workouts.

The Skinny on Your Abs

Your abs—abdominal muscles—actually comprise several different muscle groups (see the picture on page 25):

- **The rectus abdominis muscles** run vertically, from your diaphragm down to the pubic area. These are the muscles that allow you to bend forward. In very slender people with toned muscles, the rectus abdominis look like a rippling "washboard" under the skin.
- **The internal and external obliques** go from the center of your back around to the front, under the rectus abdominis. You use these muscles when you twist or bend to the side. When they're toned and tightened, they help trim your waist and flatten your abdomen.
- **The transverse abdominis muscles** are located deep under the other abdominal muscles. They surround the internal organs of the abdomen, holding them in place. Strengthening these muscles makes your midsection stronger and slimmer.

ABDOMINAL CURL (WITHOUT WEIGHTS)

When the abdominal muscles are weak—and they often are—they let it all hang out. Strengthening these muscles is like putting on an ultracomfortable twenty-four-hour girdle. The tummy and waist get tighter and trimmer—and what's more, stronger abs make for a stronger, more injury-resistant back.

Start with Level 1 Abdominal Curls. This simple move strengthens the rectus abdominis. Once that muscle gets strong, you can add a twist—Level 2—that addresses the obliques and transverse abdominis. This ingenious combination move allows you to work all of the abdominal muscle groups in a single efficient exercise.

ABDOMINAL CURL—LEVEL 1

Starting position:

Lie on your back with knees bent and feet flat on the floor. Your heels should be between 12 and 24 inches from your buttocks. Place your hands behind your ears at the base of your skull to gently support your head and neck. Focus your eyes on the ceiling.

The move:

- **1-2-3-Up:** Use your stomach muscles to slowly lift your shoulders, neck, and head one to three inches off the floor. As you get stronger, you will be able to go higher. Your eyes should stay focused on the ceiling and your chin should be slightly tucked in, but not touching your chest.
- **Pause** for a breath.
- **1-2-3-Down:** Slowly return to the starting position.
- **Pause** for a breath. Repeat.

Where you will feel the effort:

In the center of your abdomen. When this exercise is done correctly, the effort comes entirely from the abdominal muscles. You should not feel a strain in your neck. The most common cause of neck discomfort is pulling the head and neck forward during the move, or using other muscles—in your neck, shoulders, or upper back— instead of just the muscles in your abdomen.

Reps and sets:

Repeat until you have done eight abdominal curls—one set. Pause for a minute, and then do a second set.

Checklist:

- Make sure that your head is not too far forward during the lift. A good way to check: Your fist should be able to fit comfortably between your chin and upper chest.
- Move slowly.
- Don't hold your breath.
- Check for tension—and relax.

Tips:

- Think of your stomach as a sponge that is being squeezed.
- Concentrate on lifting your shoulders off the floor, not on moving your head forward.
- Imagine that you are holding an apple or orange between your chin and neck. This will help you maintain the proper position throughout the move, preventing neck strain.

ABDOMINAL CURL—LEVEL 2

Starting position:

Lie on your back with knees bent and feet flat on the floor. Your heels should be between 12 and 24 inches from your buttocks. Place your hands behind your ears at the base of your skull to gently support your head and neck. Your eyes should be focused on the ceiling.

The move:

- **1-2-3-Up:** Use your stomach muscles to slowly lift your shoulders, neck, and head two to four inches off the floor. Your eyes should stay focused on the ceiling, and your chin should be slightly tucked in, but not touching your chest. Next, gently rotate your torso to the right so that your left shoulder is reaching toward the outside of your right knee.

- **Pause** for a breath.
- **1-2-3-Down:** Return your left shoulder back to the straight position while keeping both shoulder blades lifted off of the floor two to four inches. Slowly return to the starting position.
- **Pause** for a breath, then do the same move to the opposite side, rotating your right shoulder toward your left knee.

Where you will feel the effort:

In the center of your abdomen and on both sides, along your ribs. When this exercise is done correctly, you should not feel a strain in your neck. The most common cause of neck discomfort is pulling the head and neck forward during the move or attempting to lift up higher than you can using just your abdominal muscles. Pay close attention to the position of your head and neck during the up movement and concentrate on lifting only your shoulders off the ground slightly—one to two inches—until your stomach muscles become stronger.

Reps and sets:

Repeat, alternating right and left sides. One right curl plus one left curl counts as one repetition. Do eight left-plus-right repetitions. Rest for a minute or two, and do a second set of eight reps.

Checklist:

♦ Make sure that your head is not too far forward during the Up phase. A good way to check: Your fist should be able to fit comfortably between your chin and upper chest.
♦ Move slowly.
♦ Don't hold your breath.
♦ Check for tension—and relax.

Tips:

♦ Think of your stomach as a sponge that is being squeezed.
♦ Imagine that you are holding an apple or orange between your chin and neck to prevent neck strain and to maintain proper position throughout the move.
♦ Do the Up part of the move in two distinct phases: Lift up, then rotate toward your knee.
♦ Do the Down part of the move in two distinct phases: rotate back to center, then lower.
♦ Don't let your elbow get in front of your shoulder. Your shoulder and elbow should move together, with your elbow remaining straight out to the side of your shoulder.

Pelvic Tilt (without weights)

This exercise is a classic—and for good reason. One simple move firms and strengthens your entire midsection: buttocks, thighs, abdomen, and back. It's a perfect complement to the basic program. You can do the exercise on a firm mattress or padded bench if you'd rather not get down on the floor.

Starting position:

Lie on your back with your knees bent and feet flat on the floor, shoulder-width apart. Your arms should be at your sides and relaxed, with palms flat.

The move:

- **1-2-3-Up:** Slowly roll your pelvis off the floor—first your hips, then your waist, and finally your lower back. Your midsection should form a straight line from your knees to your upper back. Your shoulders will remain on the floor.
- **Pause** for a breath.

- **1-2-3-Down:** Slowly roll back to the starting position, lowering first your back, then your waist, and finally your hips.
- **Pause** for a breath, then repeat.

Where you will feel the effort:

In the front and back of your thighs, buttocks, abdomen, and lower back.

Reps and sets:

Do eight repetitions for one set. Rest for a minute, and do another set of eight repetitions.

Checklist:

Caution: this exercise puts pressure on your upper back. If you have osteoporosis or back problems, check with your doctor before trying it.

- When you lower yourself, your movement should be controlled; don't drop onto the floor.
- Move smoothly and slowly.
- Don't hold your breath.
- Check for tension—and relax.

Tip:

If you find the move uncomfortable, don't roll quite as far back.

BACK EXTENSION (WITHOUT WEIGHTS)

Your back extensor muscles, together with the muscles in your
abdomen, serve as a protective scaffolding for the spine. This is one
of the most vulnerable parts of the body because it contains so many
joints—there's a joint between each of the twenty-four vertebrae!
The stronger your back and abdominal muscles, the less likely you
are to have pain and other back problems.

Back health is one good reason to add this exercise to your
program. The other is that it improves posture and helps you stand
taller all day long. Good posture happens to be my two-second
weight-loss program. You don't actually lose weight if you straighten
up, of course, but you can look five to ten pounds slimmer—not to
mention years younger.

Starting position:

Lie facedown on the floor on top of a folded blanket or exercise mat.
Extend your left arm over your head with your palm facing down on
the floor. Your right arm should be pointing down along the side of
your body, with your palm facing up. The tip of your nose should
touch the floor so that your neck and spine form a straight line.

The move:

♦ **1-2-3-Up:** Slowly and simultaneously lift your left arm, chest, and
  right leg off the floor approximately four to five inches. Tuck your

chin slightly to keep your head, neck, and back in line with one another.

♦ **Pause** for a breath.

♦ **1-2-3-Down:** Simultaneously lower your left arm, chest, and right leg back to the starting position in a slow and controlled manner.

♦ **Pause** for a breath, then repeat.

Where you will feel the effort:

In both your lower and upper back.

Reps and sets:

Repeat the move until you have done eight reps. Then swap arms: Move your left arm down to your side and put your right arm over your head. Do eight reps lifting your right arm and left leg. Rest for a minute, and then do a second set of eight reps on each side.

Checklist:

♦ Try to lift your upper chest off the floor while maintaining the proper positioning of your neck and head.

♦ Be sure to keep your leg as straight as possible as you lift it up.

- ◆ Move in a smooth and controlled manner off the floor as if your arm and the opposite leg were a single unit.
- ◆ Don't hold your breath.
- ◆ Check for tension—and relax.

Tip:

Look straight down as you do this exercise—this will help you maintain the proper position. Place a single paper towel on top of your mat or folded blanket as a reminder.

Push-up (without weights)

Push-ups are terrific: They strengthen several important muscle groups at once—the triceps, deltoid, pectorals, and muscles of the abdomen and back. And because you use your body weight for resistance, push-ups don't require equipment.

This is a great exercise. Yet when I suggest it, the response is often "No way!" or "Women can't do push-ups." That's not true. My mother-in-law can do twelve push-ups—and she's eighty years old.

The problem isn't anatomy but information. Few women know how to do push-ups correctly. And I must add that push-ups aren't for everyone. You'll have to skip them if you suffer from serious knee, shoulder, or back problems, or if it's hard for you to get up and down from the floor. As with any exercise, pain is a signal to back off.

It's important to do push-ups properly, and that requires a fair amount of abdominal and back strength. So if you're adding push-ups to your program, include the back and abdominal exercises as well.

Start by doing the modified push-ups—Level 1. As they become easier, graduate to Level 2. They will be difficult at first. If you can't complete two sets, do as many of the first set as you can, and then switch back to modified push-ups for the second set. Try to work up to two sets of eight Level 2 classic push-ups. Yes, that's quite a challenge. But if you persevere, you may surprise yourself.

Modified push-up—Level 1

Starting position:

Lie facedown with your palms just out to the sides of your shoulders. Your fingers will be facing forward, and your elbows will be bent and pointing up.

THE UPS AND DOWNS OF PUSH-UPS

There are two ways to do a push-up: Start Down, beginning with your torso on the floor—or Start Up, beginning with your torso raised. The choice is yours. The instructions are for Start Down.

Generally the Start Up version is harder. So instead of moving directly from Level 1 to Level 2, you can take an intermediate step from Level 1 Start Down to Level 1 Start Up. And once you master the classic push-up, you can progress to the more difficult Start Up version.

The move:

- **1-2-3-Up:** Keeping your knees on the floor, slowly push your chest up. Your body will be in an almost straight line from head to knees, with a slight bend at the hips. Stop just short of locking your elbows. Your shoulders should be above your hands.
- **Pause** for a breath.
- **1-2-3-Down:** Slowly return to the starting position.
- **Pause** for a breath. Then repeat.

Where you will feel the effort:

Shoulders, chest, and arms.

Reps and sets:

Do one set of eight repetitions. Pause for a minute, and do a second set of eight.

Checklist:

- You should feel your abdominal muscles and back muscles tighten as you do this exercise.
- Move slowly.
- Don't lock your elbows when you're in the Up position.
- Don't hold your breath.
- Check for tension—and relax.

Tip:

To make this exercise more comfortable for your knees, put a pad or rolled-up towel under them. You can also cross your ankles to take a little pressure off your knees.

CLASSIC PUSH-UP—LEVEL 2

Starting position:

Start in the same position as the modified push-up Level 1, but point your toes toward the floor.

The move:

- **1-2-3-Up:** Slowly push your body up and away from the floor, leaving only your toes and hands on the floor. Your legs, back, neck, and head should be straight. Stop just short of locking your elbows.
- **Pause** for a breath.
- **1-2-3-Down:** Return to the starting position.
- **Pause** for a breath. Repeat.

Where you will feel the effort:

Shoulder, chest, arms, and torso.

Reps and sets:

Complete eight push-ups (or as many as you can). Rest for a minute and do a second set, substituting modified push-ups if necessary.

Checklist:

◆ Keep your legs, back, and head in a straight line. You should feel your abdominal muscles and back muscles contract as you do this exercise.
◆ Move slowly.
◆ Don't lock your elbows when you're in the Up position.
◆ Don't hold your breath.
◆ Check for tension—and relax.

When you've mastered this exercise, don't be shy. Give all your friends and relatives a demonstration—and enjoy their applause.

Work toward doing this exercise from the Start Up position. Don't go all the way down when you do a Start Up push-up. At their lowest, your head, neck, and chest should be about three to four inches from the floor, but not touching, before you go back up.

SIDE ARM RAISE (WITH DUMBBELLS)

Strong, shapely shoulders look beautiful in a bathing suit or tank top. This exercise, which is also called the seated fly, really concentrates on the shoulder muscles. Stronger shoulder muscles contribute to good posture, and they help with heavy lifting.

This move takes a little practice to master, and your shoulder muscles may be weak. So use your lightest dumbbell the first time you try it. If that's too easy, move up at your next workout. If you're under age fifty, you should eventually reach eight to ten pounds; if you're fifty or over, aim for five to eight pounds.

Starting position:

Sit forward in the chair with your feet flat on the floor shoulder-width apart. With your upper arms against your sides, grasp one dumbbell in each hand, palms facing your thighs. Bend your elbows slightly. Your hands will be just in front of your hips, on the outside of your thighs.

The move:

- **1-2-3-Up:** Slowly lift your upper arms straight out to the sides, maintaining the same slight bend in your elbow. At the end of the lift, your upper arms will be parallel to the floor and straight out to the sides of your shoulders. Your forearms, still slightly bent, will also be parallel to the floor.
- **Pause** for a breath.
- **1-2-3-Down:** In a smooth motion, lower your arms back to the starting position.
- **Pause** for a breath, then repeat.

Where you will feel the effort:

In your shoulders and upper arms.

Reps and sets:

Do eight repetitions for one set. Rest for a minute, and do a second set.

Checklist:

This exercise can be confusing at first, but the move is very fluid and easy once you learn it.

- Throughout the move, keep your elbows just slightly bent. The effort should come from your shoulder muscles.
- Don't scrunch your shoulders.
- Don't let your arms come above shoulder height.
- Move slowly.
- Don't hold your breath.
- Check for tension—and relax.

▼ ▼ ▼ ▼ ▼ ▼ ▼ ▼ ▼ ▼ ▼ ▼ ▼ ▼ ▼ ▼ ▼ ▼

LUNGE (WITHOUT WEIGHTS)

The lunge is a remarkable exercise because it promotes strength, coordination, balance, and power. This move trims and tightens your lower body; it also strengthens your abs and back. In addition, you'll increase your leg power, which means you can move quickly—whether you're skiing or dodging traffic.

Unless your legs are very strong, don't attempt the lunge until you've been following this program for at least six weeks. Start with Level 1. When that is no longer challenging, progress to Level 2.

SHORT LUNGE—LEVEL 1

Starting position:

Stand to the side and back of your chair with your feet shoulder-width apart. With one hand, lightly grip the back of the chair for support.

The move:

- **1-2-3-Forward:** Take a medium step forward—about two feet—with your right leg, landing first on the heel. Your right knee should be above your right foot, but should not go past your toes. Your left knee will bend slightly, and the left heel will come up slightly off the floor.
- **Pause** for a breath.
- **Back:** Push off with your right foot to return to the starting position.
- **Pause** for a breath, then repeat, this time moving your left leg forward.

Where you will feel the effort:

In your thighs, buttocks, supporting leg, and back of ankle of supporting leg.

Reps and sets:

Repeat, alternating legs, until you have done eight lunges with each leg—that's one set. Rest for a minute, then do a second set.

Checklist:

Caution: If you have knee problems, check with your doctor before attempting the lunge.

- The toes of both feet should point straight forward throughout the movement.
- Move slowly when you go forward, but quickly when you go back.
- Don't let the leading knee go past your toes.
- Don't hold your breath.
- Check for tension—and relax. Make sure your toes are relaxed.

LUNGE—LEVEL 2

Starting position:

As in Level 1, stand to the side and back of your chair with your feet shoulder-width apart. With one hand, lightly grip the back of the chair for support.

The move:

- **1-2-3-Forward:** Take a big step forward—about three feet—with your right leg, landing first on the heel. Your right knee should be above your right foot, but should not go past your toes. Bend your left knee so it is approximately one-half of the way toward the floor. Your left heel will be off the floor.
- **Pause** for a breath.
- **Back:** Push off with your right foot to return to the starting position.
- **Pause** for a breath, then repeat, this time moving your left leg forward.

Where you will feel the effort:

In your thighs, buttocks, supporting leg, and back of the ankle of the supporting leg.

Reps and sets:

Repeat, alternating legs, until you have done eight lunges with each leg—that's one set. Rest for a minute, then do a second set.

Checklist:

- The toes of both feet should point straight forward throughout the movement.
- Move slowly when you go forward, but quickly when you go backward.
- Don't let the leading knee go past your toes.
- Don't hold your breath.
- Check for tension—and relax. Make sure your toes are relaxed.

CREATING NEW WORKOUTS

A fter you've been strength training for a few months, you'll be ready to add some or all of the new exercises. Refreshing your program helps keep you motivated—and it's good for your body. I suggest you follow your new routine for six weeks, then consider more changes to target different muscles. Over time, all your major muscles will get strong.

The chart on pages 204–05 shows six different workouts. That's just the beginning. Mix and match exercises to meet your own needs and preferences.

First, select exercises to meet your goals. Do you want to improve your posture? Work on your quadriceps to help a weak knee? Remember that certain muscle groups must be trained in pairs: If you do the knee extension, do the leg curl too; if you include the overhead press, make sure you also do either the biceps curl or the upward row; if you add the back extension, the abdominal curl should be part of the workout as well.

Then plan your new exercise routine. Workouts should be designed with safety, efficiency, and effectiveness in mind. Here are some general suggestions:

- **Begin with a warm-up:** I recommend that you keep the chair stands as your first exercise, since they not only serve as a warm-up but also train key muscle groups in the trunk and legs.
- **Next, do the exercises that require leg weights:** Beginning with the lower body helps you warm up, since you move from the large muscle groups to the smaller ones. Also, this minimizes the time you're wearing the ankle weights, which is desirable for efficiency, safety, and comfort.
- **Continue with the exercises that use dumbbells:** As you progress from large muscle groups to smaller ones, you warm your body further.
- **Do floor exercises and other exercises that don't use equipment:** Once you've finished with the equipment and put it away, it's safe to get down on the floor.
- **Cool-down and stretch:** See instructions on page 143.

For More Strengthening Exercises

See my other books—*Strong Women Stay Slim* and *Strong Women, Strong Bones*—which contain additional moves. Women who want to go further with strength training sometimes ask me to recommend sources for more exercises. Here are four excellent books:

- ◆ *A Women's Book of Strength*, by Karen Andes (Perigee, 1995).
- ◆ *Strength Training for Women*, by James A. Peterson, Ph.D. (Human Kinetics, 1995).
- ◆ *Strength Training Past 50*, by Wayne Wescott, Ph.D. (Human Kinetics, 1997).
- ◆ *The Complete Book of Butt and Legs*, by Kurt, Mike, and Brett Brungardt (Villard Books, 1995).

Also have a look at my exercise columns for *Prevention* magazine. Some are posted on the *Prevention* Web site: http://www.healthyideas.com

NEW WORKOUTS TO MEET YOUR PERSONAL GOALS

STRENGTHEN UPPER BODY	PREVENT BACK PAIN	FIRM UP ABDOMEN
I'm a runner, so my legs are in shape, but my upper body is weak.	*My back aches all the time. Sometimes it's bad enough to keep me in bed.*	*I've lost nearly thirty pounds, but I still have excess flab around my middle.*
This workout addresses the upper body and trunk, with exercises for the shoulders, arms, upper back, and abs.	Stronger back muscles help prevent back pain—and strong abs are important too. These exercises focus on the upper and lower back, plus the abs.	The best prescription is a combination of strength training and aerobic exercise (particularly walking). This workout includes key upper- and lower-body exercises plus moves aimed at toning and firming the abs.
Chair stand Biceps curl Upward row Overhead press Side arm raise Back extension Abdominal curl Pelvic tilt Push-up	Chair stand Overhead press Upward row Side arm raise Back extension Abdominal curl Pelvic tilt Lunge	Chair stand Knee extension Standing leg curl Side hip raise Upward row Overhead press Back extension Abdominal curl Pelvic tilt

New Workouts to Meet Your Personal Goals

LOOSEN TIGHT SHOULDERS	STRENGTHEN WEAK LEGS	WORK OUT WITHOUT WEIGHTS
I sit hunched over a computer all day, and my shoulders ache.	*If I walk for just fifteen minutes, I have to stop and rest my legs.*	*I need exercises I can do without equipment when I'm on the road.*
Good posture is the antidote. This workout targets postural and upper back muscles.	These exercises will increase strength in the legs and trunk and add power to the legs.	This efficient workout addresses most of the major muscle groups— without weights.
Chair stand Upward row Overhead press Side arm raise Back extension Abdominal curl Pelvic tilt Push-up	Chair stand Knee extension Standing leg curl Side hip raise Back extension Abdominal curl Pelvic tilt Lunge Toe stand	Chair stand Back extension Abdominal curl Pelvic tilt Push-up Lunge Toe stand

◆ ◆ ◆

The unforeseen benefits of strength training have been extra-ordinary. I find I am standing taller, not because I have to re-mind myself, but because my body is reacting to becoming stronger as I work the muscles in various areas. My mindset has changed—I remind myself that if I can lift these weights, I can do so many other things. I do volunteer work at our provincial archives, a walk of about twenty-five minutes each way. Yesterday was a glorious summer morning. I was actually strutting along, feeling so powerful and well. As I walked past an outdoor bagel shop, I saw a man do a double take as I passed his table. That was quite a moment for this seventy-three-year-old woman!
—*Olive*

I was one hundred pounds overweight and had high blood pres-sure and cholesterol. I went immediately to the book store and bought it. I read the book, got the weights and started. Within six weeks of changing my eating habits, exercising every day (three of those days with weights), I lost twenty-one pounds. My doctor checked my blood pressure and it was absolutely nor-mal. I cried at that appointment! I was and still am very happy.
—*Laurie*

◆ ◆ ◆

DOING THE PROGRAM AT A GYM

When my *JAMA* study was published, I received hundreds of calls and letters from women all around the world who wanted strength-training exercises that were cheap and easy to do at home. That's why the program in this book uses free weights—dumbbells and ankle cuffs.

But I also heard from women who wanted to know how to strength-train on weight-lifting machines at a health club. And that's why I'm including this chapter. As you'll see, it doesn't merely duplicate the at-home program. Instead, I've put together the best possible workout you can do in about forty minutes on strength-training machines.

Which version is better—home or fitness center?

Both programs will make you stronger. *The best version is the one you prefer,* because that's the one you're more likely to do. I use both. I have free weights at home and train on the machines at work.

HEALTH CLUB, FITNESS CENTER, GYM— WHAT'S THE DIFFERENCE?

I use these terms interchangeably because there's no generally accepted distinction. Usually, though, a health club provides more than just exercise; for instance, it might have massage, nutrition counseling, or health-related classes. But some fitness centers offer these, too. The word *gym* is the most general and covers everything from the simplest exercise area in a local high school to a luxurious facility with ultramodern equipment and extensive services.

WHY JOIN A FITNESS CENTER?

Here are some of the pluses:

◆ YOU CAN STRENGTH-TRAIN ON MACHINES INSTEAD OF (OR ALONG WITH) FREE WEIGHTS

Machines are designed to get you into the right position for a move. This means you can isolate the muscle you're working without having to pay quite as much attention to the rest of your body. As a result, most people can work out at a higher intensity than they can with free weights. That can be an important advantage for women concerned about osteoporosis, who want to stimulate their bones as much as possible.

Jayne liked the convenience of strength training at home, but after a few months, she joined a gym so she could use machines. She explains:

I have arthritic knees, and it hurts to stand on one foot. Even though I knew the leg exercises were particularly important for me, some were uncomfortable to do with free weights. And I can't get down on the floor for back and abdominal exercises. With the machines, I can do all the exercises sitting down, which is much more comfortable.

◆ INSTRUCTION IS USUALLY AVAILABLE

A fitness trainer can fine-tune your workouts and get you past any rough spots.

◆ YOU'RE NOT ALONE

Other people provide companionship, advice, and encouragement. Bonnie, a member of the nonexercise group in my *JAMA* study, decided to join a gym to get in shape after the project was over. She found inspiration in the changing room:

I met a woman who was training for a bodybuilding contest. I thought she was about twenty-eight years old—but she was forty-five and had been heavy. She told me that one day she saw a program on Oprah *about women who had lost weight, and she decided to join a diet group and work out. I thought: "If she could do that, so can I."*

◆ FITNESS FACILITIES HAVE OTHER EXERCISE EQUIPMENT

As you get stronger, you might enjoy using treadmills, stair climbers, or rowers. Such facilities may offer classes such as step aerobics or tai chi. Anything that encourages you to become more active is an advantage. Jayne's knee problems rule out a walking program and most sports. She comments:

At the health club, they have machines I can use for an aerobic workout. For instance, there's a recumbent stair climber. You lie on your back on this slanted platform that goes from your head to your hips, and you push huge pedals up and down with your legs. It looks ridiculous, but boy, do I sweat.

◆ HEALTH CLUBS MAY OFFER ADDITIONAL SERVICES

They may have nutrition classes or massage or other features that you find appealing.

HOW TO SELECT A FITNESS CENTER

Health clubs have transformed themselves in the past decade. Don't assume they're just for jocks and Lycra-clad women with perfect bodies! Go have a look. You may be surprised to find people of all physical types, with muscular young men working out side by side with elderly women, and special classes for the fat and the frail as well as the already fit.

If you want to explore this option, start by listing the facilities near your home, your work, or some other place you visit at least three or four times a week. Think very carefully before joining a club that's more than fifteen or twenty minutes away. No matter how wonderful a fitness center is, if it's not convenient, most women don't continue using it. Check your Yellow Pages under "Health Clubs" or "Exercise and Physical Fitness Programs." If you live near a school or college, call and ask if its facilities are available to people in the neighborhood. Also find out if your local community center or Y has a gym. By the way, many Y's are now upscale, with superb staff and equipment.

You can narrow down the possibilities on the phone by asking a few simple questions. Inquire about hours and whether a place has the facilities and programs you want. If money is a deciding factor, find out about costs. You can then request a brochure, or make an appointment to visit and talk to the manager.

What to Look For

There's no substitute for a tour of the club. Schedule your visit for the same time of day you'd be there to work out—that's the best way to learn if conditions are likely to be crowded. Look at the exercise floor, of course, but also check out the changing room, read the notices on the bulletin board, and visit any areas you expect to use, such as the pool or child-care facility. Use your nose and ears as well as your eyes; a health club shouldn't smell bad, and the noise level should be acceptable.

Ask yourself:

- **Is everything clean and well lit?** Don't forget to peek into the rest rooms.
- **What kind of equipment is used?** The three top brands of strength-training machines are Keiser, Nautilus, and Cybex. Other good lines are made by Body Master and Life Fitness.
- **Is the equipment in good repair?** While you can't always be sure, causes for concern include: Not Working signs on machines; frayed cables; ripped seats; creaking noises that sound as if equipment is not well maintained. (The same advice applies if you're checking out a fitness room at a hotel, an office, or an apartment house.)
- **Will the machines fit you?** Petite women, especially, need to check. Though this is changing, equipment sometimes is designed for men and can't easily be adjusted to fit a smaller-than-average woman.
- **How many staff members are on the floor?** Optimally, at least one trainer will supervise each exercise area—more at busy times. When you have a question, you shouldn't have to stop your workout and go searching for a trainer; nor should you be forced to wait in a long line because there aren't enough instructors to respond to members.
- **Are instructors attentive?** I've seen gyms where a third of the people working out are doing something incorrect or

even unsafe—but the instructors are just standing around chatting with each other. This reflects poor training and supervision.

♦ **Is the equipment available?** Or are there lines and long waits for popular machines?

♦ **Is there enough space between machines?** You don't want to be elbow-to-elbow with other exercisers.

♦ **Is the ambience right for you?** Is this a place you'll be glad to come to? Are there people similar to you in age and level of fitness? Do you prefer a coed facility or one that's just for women?

Questions to Ask

You'll learn a lot from your own observations, but other important information won't be so obvious. The director or another staff member can answer these questions:

♦ **What kind of programming do you offer?** If you've just had a baby, ask if there are postpartum programs; if you're a senior, ask about activities for older exercisers.

♦ **What trade organizations do you belong to?** Many high-end health clubs are members of IHRSA—the International Health, Racquet & Sports Club Association. (Some excellent clubs don't participate in this organization, however.)

♦ **What qualifications do staff members have? How long have they worked here, on average?** For safety, all should be CPR certified. Ideally, the professional staff—instructors, physical therapists, dietitians—should have the appropriate credentials in their specialties. (Organizations that certify fitness trainers are listed on page 215.) There's a lot of turnover in this field, but it will be better if you see mostly the same faces every month.

- **How long have you been in business?** Unfortunately, many fitness centers open and quickly close. I suggest you pick one that's been around for at least a couple of years.
- **What is the fee?** A good club will give you the option of an introductory membership, which usually lasts four to six weeks. Sad to say, a few fitness centers have given the entire business an unsavory reputation for high-pressure sales tactics. You may be told if you join that day, they'll waive the initiation fee. Try to persuade the salesperson to extend the offer, so you don't have to decide on the spot. Before you make a commitment, call your local Better Business Bureau to see if there have been any complaints about a facility you're considering.

The International Health, Racquet & Sports Club Association will mail you a free brochure, *How to Choose a Quality Club,* if you send a request with a stamped, self-addressed business-size envelope to IHRSA, 263 Summer Street, Boston, MA 02210.

WORKING WITH A FITNESS TRAINER

When you join a health club, you'll have access to a fitness trainer on the exercise floor. Your membership also may include a limited number of private or group training sessions. This is an excellent benefit, and I urge you to take advantage of it—especially if you have special needs or concerns.

A good trainer can do a lot for you:

- When you begin the program, the trainer will show you how to use the equipment correctly.
- The trainer can check your form and answer questions as you learn the exercises.
- The trainer can offer encouragement and help solve any problems that come up.

The terminology for different kinds of trainers is still evolving, but most people in the field make the following distinction:

Fitness trainers, also called **fitness instructors,** are gym staff members who are available on the exercise floor. They're knowledgeable about exercise and know how to use the machines.

Personal trainers work with you as an individual. Sometimes they're hired through a gym, nearly always for an extra fee. You also can arrange for a trainer to come to your home or office. Good personal trainers have more training and experience than most fitness instructors, though the same individual may serve in both capacities.

♦ As your needs change, the trainer can help you adjust the program.

The amount of personal instruction you get from the fitness trainers at your gym depends on the nature of the club and your membership agreement. Not surprisingly, the more expensive the club, the more individual attention you're likely to receive.

To maximize access to your gym's trainers, try to work out at an off-peak hour when fewer members need help. Don't be shy about asking for assistance! A good trainer wants you to succeed and will be glad to work with you.

Hiring a Personal Trainer

You may get everything you need from the fitness trainers at your gym. But if you want more individual attention, you can hire a personal trainer to work with you one-on-one. Many fitness centers offer this service for an additional fee. A personal trainer also could be very helpful if you're working out at home or at a gym that doesn't have instructors.

HOW DO YOU KNOW IF A TRAINER IS QUALIFIED?

At the time this book was written and revised, personal trainers weren't licensed in any state, but the situation may change. Anyone can call himself or herself a personal trainer—and tens of thousands do. How do you find someone with good education and experience? The easiest way is to look for a trainer who's certified by a reputable program. There are hundreds of such programs, but the following seven are best if you want a person knowledgeable about strength training.

- **American College of Sports Medicine:** ACSM is an established organization with more than fifteen thousand members in over fifty countries. Its activities include scientific research as well as training. I'm a fellow of ACSM and am certified by them as a health fitness director.
- **National Strength and Conditioning Association**
- **National Academy of Sports Medicine (NASM)**
- **American Council on Exercise (ACE)**
- **Aerobics and Fitness Association of America (AFAA)**
- **International Association of Fitness Professionals (IDEA)**
- **Cooper Institute for Aerobics Research**

When you contact a trainer, ask for a brochure or other written materials. Then check for appropriate certification. Most personal trainers have certification from at least one of these organizations; fitness instructors usually have just a single certification.

Deciding if a Trainer Is Right for You

It takes more than certification to make a great teacher—you know that from school. The same is true of trainers: The best person is the one whose skills match your needs. The trainer I'd recommend for an Olympic-caliber marathon runner isn't the one I'd suggest to an out-of-shape forty-seven-year-old woman who wants to start strength training.

Here are some issues to consider, both before you select a personal trainer and as you continue working together:

- Does the trainer have experience helping people like you?
- Does the trainer understand and share your goals for yourself?
- Do you understand the trainer's instructions? Do they make sense to you?
- When the trainer corrects you, do you feel helped rather than criticized?
- Do you feel comfortable asking questions?
- Do you look forward to your sessions with the trainer? Do you feel good about yourself afterward?
- Does the trainer focus on your exercise program rather than attempt to sell you additional products and services?
- Is the trainer able to adapt the program as your needs change?
- Do you feel you're progressing and meeting your goals?

What About Costs?

You don't have to be a movie star to hire a personal trainer! Expect to pay from under $50 per hour, if you make arrangements through your gym, to $75 to $100 per hour, if the trainer comes to your home. And for a trainer who caters to the rich and famous, fees start at $200 per hour.

A few money-saving possibilities:

- Inquire about a discount for multiple sessions, if you know you'll want to see the trainer at least six times.

- Ask whether the trainer will let you form a mini-class, then recruit a few friends to work out with you and split the fee.
- See the trainer only at a few key times—when you're learning the exercises, if you run into trouble, or every six months for a checkup.

STRENGTH TRAINING ON MACHINES

Much of what you've learned from this book—how lifting weights affects your body, how to motivate yourself for positive change, how to stay on track—applies to any strength-training program, regardless of what equipment you use. The specific exercises are different, however. The gym version of my program consists of ten exercises—nine done on machines, plus the toe stands from the at-home version. Together they strengthen the major muscle groups in your arms, legs, back, and abdomen.

The instructions below are general because it's beyond the scope of this book to describe all available machines. **Before you begin, you will need to work closely with a fitness instructor or personal trainer to learn how to use the equipment properly.**

Getting Started

Make an appointment for one or two sessions with a trainer. Explain that you'd like to follow this program and need assistance to start. Here's what these sessions should cover:

♦ WHAT EQUIPMENT TO USE

If the facility doesn't have the machines recommended here—or if the available machines don't fit you properly—ask the instructor to suggest substitute exercises. Plan a program that's convenient for the particular layout of the gym. In general, I suggest alternating leg and upper-body exercises to avoid fatigue, but this isn't essential.

◆ How to Position Yourself and Make the Move

Because exercise machines are designed to keep you in position, it's very important to set the seat, the pads, and other adjustable elements to line up correctly with your body. Write down the settings to be sure you remember them! *Don't ever hesitate to ask questions if you aren't certain how to perform an exercise safely and effectively.*

◆ How and at What Level to Set the Resistance

The instructor will teach you how to set the resistance. If you're using weight stacks that go up by ten- to twenty-pound increments, ask how to use special two-and-a-half- and five-pound add-on weights to make the increases smoother as you get stronger.

The resistance settings on exercise machines may be described as "pounds" or "kilograms," *but they don't necessarily correspond to the pounds of free weights.* This means you'll have to rely on the Exercise Intensity Scale (page 151), along with your instructor's advice, to decide where to start, how fast to progress, and when you've reached a good level to maintain.

DON'T FORGET TO KEEP LOGS!

Nearly all fitness centers provide logs because it's so important to keep careful records. The machines you're using will be set up for the previous user, not you. Your log enables you to adjust the seat, the resistance, and other settings as accurately and efficiently as possible. And, of course, your log is a terrific source of motivation.

General Instructions for Each Session

As with free weights, you'll train twice a week, allowing at least one day between sessions. Here are some guidelines.

- ◆ Warm-up: Do five minutes of light aerobic activity to get your body warm and ready for the exercises.
- ◆ Perform the exercises slowly, with a three-second rest between repetitions.
- ◆ Take a one-minute rest between sets.
- ◆ Do two sets of eight repetitions of each exercise.
- ◆ Cool-down and stretch.

Do not attempt to exercise on strength-training machines until you've been shown how to use them correctly.

WHEN YOU'RE AWAY FROM YOUR GYM

Dorothy—the grandmother of seventeen who joined a Y after her year in our study—likes to work out wherever she travels. She says:

If there's a Y, I can use my membership there. Otherwise I look up "Fitness Centers" in the phone book and ask if they'll let me come in on a day rate. One time I was setting up the leg press next to a young fellow who was working on another machine. He must have thought the little old lady needed help, because he offered to do it for me. He was quite surprised when I told him the setting.

KNEE EXTENSION

This is the machine version of the knee extension in the at-home program—the move that shapes your quadriceps (front thigh muscles) and adds power to your walk.

- **Position yourself:** Adjust the backrest so your knees are just over the edge of the seat. The center part of your knee joint should be aligned with the joint of the machine, so both bend together. Adjust the roller pads in front of your shins, just above your ankle joint. The pads should *not* rest on the tops of your feet. Unfortunately, many older machines are difficult to adjust to smaller women. Ask the trainer to help you make the best possible adjustment.
- **Set the resistance.**
- **Lightly grasp the handholds,** or rest your hands on your thighs.
- **1-2-3-Up:** Slowly extend your lower legs so your knees go from a ninety-degree angle to being as straight as possible.
- **Pause** for a breath.
- **1-2-3-Down:** Slowly lower your legs to the starting position.
- **Pause** for a breath.

Reps and sets:

Repeat for a total of eight times for one set. Rest for a minute, and do a second set of eight repetitions.

Checklist:

- Don't grip the handholds tightly—when you use extra muscle groups, your quadriceps get less of a workout.
- To get the full benefit from this exercise, it's important to extend your legs as straight as possible. If you can't extend your legs completely, lower the resistance to allow the fullest possible extension. As you get stronger and more flexible, your range of motion will increase.
- If you have an orthopedic problem in one of your knees and the strength of your two legs is very uneven, train one leg at a time. This enables you to adjust the resistance to each leg.
- Don't hold your breath.
- Check for tension—and relax.

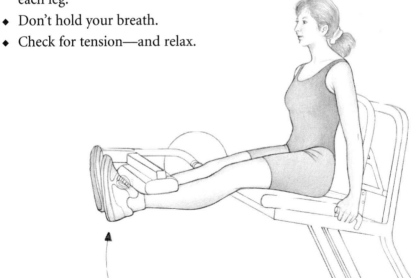

OVERHEAD PRESS

This exercise corresponds to the overhead press in Chapter 8. It works the triceps in back of your upper arms, giving you strength for over-the-head tasks—as well as the deltoid and trapezius muscles of your upper back, which keep you standing tall.

- **Position yourself:** Adjust the seat height so the arm handles are at the same level as your shoulders. Place your back firmly and comfortably against the backrest.
- **Set the resistance.**
- **Grasp the handles** with palms facing forward.

- **1-2-3-Up:** Slowly raise your arms up over your head until they are fully extended.
- **Pause** for a breath.
- **1-2-3-Down:** Slowly return to the starting position.
- **Pause** for a breath.

Reps and sets:

Repeat for a total of eight times for one set. Rest for a minute, and do a second set of eight repetitions.

Checklist:

- Your back should remain against the cushion throughout the lift.
- Maintain good posture.
- Don't hold your breath.
- Check for tension—and relax.

DOUBLE LEG PRESS

This exercise is a real fanny firmer. It works the muscles in your buttocks (gluteus maximus) and your quadriceps. You'll see a difference in any activity that uses your legs.

Caution: Don't use a double leg press machine that positions you lying down with your shoulders up against pads. This position puts a lot of pressure on the spine and shoulders—not a good idea, especially for older women or anyone with back problems.

- **Position yourself:** Sit in the seat, and place your feet in the middle of the foot pads in front of you. Adjust the seat close enough to the foot pads so your knees form a ninety-degree angle. If ninety degrees is uncomfortable, move the seat back to straighten your legs a little. As you become stronger and more flexible, work toward moving the seat forward and having your knees at a ninety-degree angle.
- **Set the resistance.**
- **Lightly grasp the handles.**

- **1-2-3-Out:** Slowly push your legs so the foot pads move away from your body and your knees are just short of being fully extended. **Don't lock your knees at the end of the move.** That would strain the knee joints.
- **Pause** for a breath.
- **1-2-3-Back:** Slowly return to the starting position.
- **Pause** for a breath.

Reps and sets:

Repeat for a total of eight times for one set. Rest for a minute, and do a second set of eight repetitions.

Checklist:

- If you have an orthopedic problem in one hip or knee and your legs are very uneven in strength, you can do this exercise with one leg at a time. This will let you adjust the resistance to the proper intensity for each leg.
  - Don't forget to breathe.
  - Check for tension—and relax.

FRONT LATERAL PULL-DOWN

Nothing makes you look older than bad posture. This exercise—which gives the biceps and back muscles (rhomboid and latissimus dorsi) a workout—helps prevent slumping. In addition, lateral pull-downs strengthen the bones in the spine. I wish I could have included this exercise in the at-home program, because it's such an excellent choice for women. Unfortunately, there's no free-weight version (though women who are already very fit can use a chin-up bar at home).

- **Position yourself:** Sit down facing the machine, with your feet flat on the floor. Adjust the seat height so that your arms will be fully extended, but the elbows not locked, when you reach up to grasp the ends of the bar. Adjust the pad so it rests snugly on top of your thighs, to stabilize your lower body.
- **Set the resistance.**
- **Grasp the bar** over your head with an overhand closed grip: your thumb and fingers should wrap around the bar completely, with your palms facing forward. Your hands should be slightly wider than shoulder-width apart, so your arms form a wide *V*. Lean back slightly from the hips so that the bar is directly over your chest. Squeeze your shoulder blades together.

- **1-2-3-Down:** Slowly bend your elbows down and toward your sides, to pull the bar down in front of your head until it is just above your collarbone.
- **Pause** for a breath.
- **1-2-3-Up:** Slowly return to the starting position, with your arms fully extended overhead.
- **Pause** for a breath.

Reps and sets:

Repeat for a total of eight times for one set. Rest for a minute, and do a second set of eight reps.

Checklist:

- To get the full benefit of this exercise, you must move the bar through a full range of motion—from the starting position over your head down to the base of your neck, just above the collarbone.
- Be sure to maintain your body position: Don't bend or move your torso, or let your lower back collapse as you lower the bar.
- Check the position of your hands to be sure they're the same distance from the ends of the bar.
- Don't hold your breath.
- Check for tension—and relax.

Leg Curl

This exercise (like the standing leg curl in the at-home program) works your hamstrings, the muscles in the back of your thighs, making them more shapely. If vanity isn't a motivator, consider that the hamstrings are the partner muscles to the quadriceps. So it's important to train them as you train the quads to keep them in balance.

Note: I've described seated leg curls. The same exercise is also done on a machine that positions you lying on your stomach. Both versions are fine, although the seated version minimizes the stress on your lower back.

- **Position yourself:** Adjust the backrest so your knees are just over the edge of the seat. Your knee joint should be aligned with the joint of the machine so the two bend together. Place the thigh pads snugly over your thighs and the ankle pads under your ankles, just above the joints. These devices hold your legs comfortably in place as you

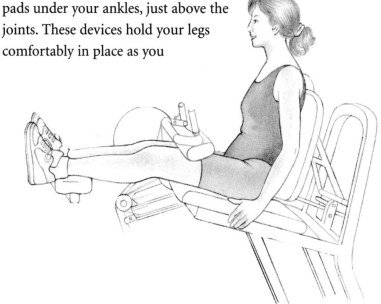

do the exercise. Your knees should be just slightly bent, not straight and locked.

- **Set the resistance.**
- **Lightly grasp the handholds.**
- **1-2-3-Down:** Slowly bend your knees until they are at a ninety-degree angle.
- **Pause** for a breath.
- **1-2-3-Back:** Slowly return to the starting position.
- **Pause** for a breath.

Reps and sets:

Repeat for a total of eight times for one set. Rest for a minute, and do a second set of eight repetitions.

Checklist:

- If the pads are uncomfortable, ask the fitness trainer to help you adjust them.
- Don't hold your breath.
- Check for tension—and relax.

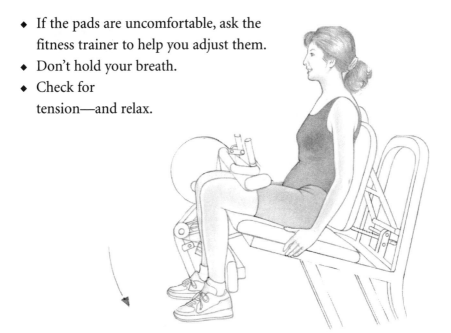

BICEPS CURL

This exercise corresponds to the biceps curl done with dumbbells in the at-home version of the program. Either way, the move tones your upper arms and strengthens the biceps—muscles you rely on every time you raise your arm.

- **Position yourself:** Adjust the seat height so the backs of your arms rest comfortably over the arm cushions in front of you.
- **Set the resistance.**
- **Extend your arms straight forward,** resting the backs of your upper arms on the pads. Grasp the hand grips with your palms facing up. Make sure the joint on the arm of the machine is directly in line with your elbow joints so they bend together.

- **1-2-3-Up:** Slowly contract your biceps muscles to bring your hands up toward your shoulders. Your arms should bend *only* at the elbows; the backs of your upper arms should remain on the pads throughout the exercise.
- **Pause** for a breath.
- **1-2-3-Down:** Slowly return to the starting position.
- **Pause** for a breath.

Reps and sets:

Repeat for a total of eight times for one set. Rest for a minute, and do a second set of eight repetitions.

Checklist:

- Your elbows are the only joints that should move when you do this exercise; your shoulders and the rest of your body should remain still.
- Maintain good posture as you make the move.
- Don't hold your breath.
- Check for tension—and relax.

SEATED ROW

This exercise strengthens the muscles of the upper-middle back, which helps to improve posture. If you spend the day hunched over a desk—and are feeling the effects in your neck, shoulders, and upper back—here's the perfect antidote.

- **Position yourself:** Sit facing the machine with your feet flat on the floor. Adjust the seat height first: Your arms should be parallel to the floor when you reach straight forward to touch the handles. Then adjust the chest pad so that the top is in line with your upper chest.
- **Set the resistance.**
- **Grasp the handles** with a closed grip—your thumb and fingers should wrap around the handles completely. Your palms should face each other.
- **1-2-3-Down:** Slowly pull the handles back toward your body, until your elbows pass your sides. Your upper arm and forearm should form a right angle.
- **Pause** for a breath.
- **1-2-3-Up:** Slowly return to the starting position, with your arms fully extended.
- **Pause** for a breath.

Reps and sets:

Repeat for a total of eight times for one set. Rest for a minute, and do a second set of eight reps.

Checklist:

- Keep your chest lightly pressed against the pad throughout the move. This will help you maintain the correct position. Do not let your chest pull away from the pad as you move your arms back.
- Keep your head up with your eyes focused forward. Don't let your chin drop toward your chest.
- Keep your elbows next to your ribs as you pull your arms back.
- Don't hold your breath.
- Check for tension—and relax.

▼ ▼ ▼ ▼ ▼ ▼ ▼ ▼ ▼ ▼ ▼ ▼ ▼ ▼ ▼ ▼ ▼ ▼

Back Extension

Good posture makes you stand taller—so you look younger, slimmer, and more confident. This exercise strengthens the back extensor muscles, which will make it easier for you to maintain good posture all day. On the more functional side, a stronger back is less vulnerable to injuries, even if you carry heavy objects. And there's a bone bonus: This exercise helps maintain the bones of your spine. Though you can work the same muscles with the supplemental back exercises in Chapter 11, the machine version doesn't require that you get down on the floor.

Note: If you have back problems or have injured your back in the past, check with your health care provider to make sure this exercise is safe for you.

- **Position yourself:** Sit with your back against the seat back, facing forward. Snugly fasten the seat belt or other stabilizing device. (If the machine doesn't have one, don't do the exercise—it would be very difficult to perform the move properly.)
- **Set the resistance.**
- **Grasp the handholds,** or cross your hands across your chest.
- **1-2-3-Out:** Slowly extend your torso back, while keeping your head perpendicular to the floor. This means that as you lean back, your chin will tip slightly toward your chest.

- **Pause** for a breath.
- **1-2-3-Back:** Slowly return to the starting position.
- **Pause** for a breath.

Reps and sets:

Repeat for a total of eight times for one set. Rest for a minute, and do a second set of eight repetitions.

Checklist:

- Don't be concerned if you need to set the resistance much lower than others at the gym. Most people don't do this exercise properly: Instead of relying on their back muscles, they use their leg muscles to push against the foot plate and move their torso back. While this allows them to move a lot of weight, they aren't strengthening their back.
- Most women have weak back extensor muscles, so it's important to progress slowly on this exercise.
- To stabilize your neck and head, focus on a spot at eye level on the wall in front of you when you're in the starting position, and maintain that focus throughout the exercise.
- Don't hold your breath.
- Check for tension—and relax.

ABDOMINAL CURL

If you want a flat, firm stomach, this exercise is for you. Also your abdominal muscles, together with the back extensors, help stabilize and protect your spine. The abdominal exercises in Chapter 11 provide the same benefits but are done on the floor.

Caution: If you have back problems, or if you have osteoporosis, check with your health care provider to make sure this exercise is safe and appropriate.

- **Position yourself:** Adjust the seat height so the chest pads fit comfortably on your upper chest—above your breasts and below the bony part of your collarbone.
- **Set the resistance.**
- **Lightly grasp the handhold.** You want your abdominal muscles to do all the work, so don't use your hands to help.

- **1-2-3-Down:** Slowly squeeze your stomach muscles so your shoulders come closer to your hips. When you do this exercise properly, your shoulders will move only about two to three inches. If you're going farther, ask the fitness trainer for instructions. You may be using hip muscles, not your abdominals—and that could injure your back.
- **Pause** for a breath.
- **1-2-3-Back:** Return to the starting position.
- **Pause** for a breath.

Reps and sets:

Repeat for a total of eight times for one set. Rest for a minute, and do a second set of eight repetitions.

Checklist:

- To get the feel of the exercise before you do it for the first time, sit in a chair and slowly squeeze your stomach muscles so your shoulders come closer to your hips. (It may help to imagine that your stomach is being squeezed like a sponge.) You will see that you don't bend forward very much when you contract your abdominal muscles.
- Don't forget to breathe.
- Check for tension—and relax.

▼ ▼ ▼ ▼ ▼ ▼ ▼ ▼ ▼ ▼ ▼ ▼ ▼ ▼ ▼ ▼ ▼

TOE STAND

This is the same exercise used in the at-home program (see page 139). While you could work the same muscles on gym equipment, you'd be seated and stabilized. So, you wouldn't receive the added benefit of improving your balance and coordination that you get from the toe stand.

HOW TO PROGRESS

Follow the basic principles set out in Chapter 9, along with the advice of your instructor, to devise an individual program.

- During the first few sessions, when you're learning to use the equipment, set the machines so that you are working at Level 3 on the Exercise Intensity Scale—lifting the weight is well within your capability but would tire you if continued for a long time.
- By the second or third week, increase the weight so you're working at Level 4—you can do the move eight times in good form, but after that you need to rest. During the first twelve weeks, you should try to increase the load every week or two. But don't attempt to advance more quickly, since you'll be lifting heavier weights with the machine than you would with free weights.
- As you get stronger and less effort is needed, increase the weight to maintain Level 4 intensity.
- After you've been training for six months to a year, progress is likely to become much slower. Ask your instructor about adding or swapping new exercises.

WHEN YOU'RE READY FOR MORE

I've chosen these ten exercises because they provide an excellent overall strengthening workout in about forty minutes. After you've been doing them for a month or two, you may want to expand your activities. Great! That's what gym membership is all about. Consider taking an aerobics or yoga class; experiment with machines you haven't tried before. I encourage you to discuss the possibilities with your instructor.

You can add new strengthening exercises to vary your workout or target other muscle groups. Here are a few of my other favorites:

- Hip abduction: Exercise your outer thigh muscles—the same ones worked by the side hip raise from the basic program.
- Hip adduction: This exercise, which works the inner thighs, complements the hip abduction.
- Flies: This exercise strengthens the front of your shoulders and your upper chest muscles, which will firm your bosom.

MEN NEED STRENGTH TRAINING TOO!

◆ ◆ ◆

I was a tennis teaching pro until ten years ago, when I turned sixty and developed arthritis in my left knee. At first I could still play if I took pain medication, but after about four years I had to stop playing tennis altogether. As of last year, it was hard to walk without caving in to pain. Even getting up from a chair hurt a lot. Then I started a Tufts strength-training program.

Within three months I started playing tennis again. Four months later, I flew to California to play in the United States Professional Tennis Championships—and I placed number two in the seventy-to-seventy-five-year-old category! I want to keep playing tennis into my nineties.

—Al

If I'm in a bad mood, I go to the gym and lift weights. That always gets me out of the slump. After a workout, my body feels more alive. And somehow I feel more content with life.
—Sam

◆　◆　◆

Men typically have more muscle and stronger bones than women do. But they also lose strength, bone mass, and balancing ability as they get older. Beginning around age thirty, men lose about 1 percent of their muscle strength each year. The change accelerates to about 2 percent per year after age sixty. By the time a man reaches his eightieth birthday, typically he's lost about 60 percent of the strength he had at age thirty.

Thanks to their head start, men take longer to reach the danger point. But if they live long enough, they too are at risk for frailty, falls, and fractures. Fortunately, strength training can help. Men benefit in the same ways that women do. Indeed, studies at Tufts and elsewhere have found that when men and women follow the very same exercise program, men gain about 30 percent more muscle mass.

The exercises in this book work just as well for men as they do for women. The only difference is that men can start with weights that are one or two pounds heavier, and they can expect to reach higher goals.

Here's how to adapt the *Strong Women* program if you're a man:

◆ YOUR STARTING POINT

Answer the questions on pages 147 to 148. Then use the table on the next page, designed for men, instead of the table on page 148.

◆ THE EXERCISES

Follow the instructions in the book. Begin the program with the basic eight exercises, adding moves from Chapter 11 when you're ready for them. Do the exercises twice a week, with at least one day of rest between workouts. Use the same guidelines to advance: Select a weight that you can lift eight times in good form—but not much more than that—before your

Osteoporosis Isn't Just a Women's Disease

Many men are astonished to learn that they can develop osteoporosis and suffer hip fractures. In fact, it's a common problem. Two million American men have osteoporosis. Each year, 100,000 men fracture a hip. Despite these alarming numbers, male osteoporosis often goes undiagnosed because men—and even doctors—think of it as a problem that only women have.

muscles need to rest. As you get stronger, increase the weight to maintain the same level of effort.

STARTING LEVEL FOR MEN	POUNDS FOR EACH ARM	POUNDS FOR EACH LEG
Beginning	2	3
Intermediate	3	4
Advanced	5	6

STRENGTH-TRAINING GOALS FOR MEN
(POUNDS AND LEVELS)

EXERCISE	AGE 49 AND YOUNGER	AGE 50 TO 69	AGE 70 AND OLDER
Standing leg curl	15 to 18	12 to 18	8 to 16
Knee extension	18 to 20	12 to 18	10 to 18
Side hip raise	15 to 18	12 to 18	8 to 16
Biceps curl	20 to 25	15 to 20	10 to 20
Overhead press	15 to 20	12 to 18	10 to 15
Upward row	20 to 25	15 to 20	12 to 20
Toe stand	Level 2	Level 2	Level 2
Side arm raise (supplemental)	12 to 15	8 to 12	8 to 12

♦ GOALS

Most men eventually reach levels that are 25 to 50 percent higher than those reached by women the same age. The table above (which corresponds to the table for women on page 157) presents goals for men. Don't regard them as upper limits—you may advance even further. But heed the same caution I give women: Don't go above twenty pounds with the ankle weights or above twenty-five pounds with dumbbells, since heavier versions could become a problem for your joints.

◆ ◆ ◆

I've always been active—swimming, walking, and playing tennis—but nagging knee pain and weakness in my legs were compromising the sports and hobbies I enjoy most. I had developed a mild limp. Then I started a structured strength-training program. Within just a couple of months, I was feeling noticeably better. Now, less than a year later, my knee pain has almost completely disappeared, something I never dreamed possible. The limp is gone. Going on walks in the woods is easier. The uneven terrain that was once challenging and difficult is enjoyable again. I feel confident that I can maintain the tremendous gains I've achieved and continue to enjoy life to the fullest.
—John

I'm forty-three. I don't look or feel very different from the way I looked and felt in my twenties. But every so often, I get a powerful reminder that things have changed. A few months ago, I was making a hay fort with my kids, throwing around fifty-pound bales of hay. After about twenty minutes of this, I picked up a bale—and pain shot through my elbow and down my forearm. It took me completely by surprise. I was in pain for twenty-four hours. After I recovered, I added arm exercises to my strength-training routine to build up the muscles around my elbows.

I'm learning that my body now needs a lot more maintenance for me to keep doing the physical activities I've always enjoyed. I don't think of strength training as a wonder drug. It's more like brushing and flossing my teeth.
—Sam

◆ ◆ ◆

QUESTIONS &
ANSWERS

've tried to anticipate your questions throughout the text. But if I missed something, I hope you'll find the answer here.

GENERAL QUESTIONS ABOUT
STRENGTH TRAINING

Q: Can this program help me lose weight?

A: Yes. Strength training—along with cutting calories and doing aerobic exercise—is a terrific way to lose fat as well as pounds. The more muscle you have, the higher your metabolic rate. This means that when you add strength training to your weight-loss program, you can eat a little more. Also, if you've been dieting and have reached a plateau, strength training could help you move past it. Strength training also helps indirectly because it makes aerobic activity more enjoyable.

LIFT WEIGHTS, LOSE WEIGHT

Strength training is a super way to power weight loss. It not only helps take off pounds, it also trims and tightens. For detailed instructions, see my second book, *Strong Women Stay Slim,* or do the following:

- Adjust your food intake so you lose weight gradually, at a rate of no more than two pounds a week. Women who try to speed the process usually lose muscle as well as fat and get fewer nutrients, and what's more, they feel deprived and risk regaining the weight later on.
- Do strength training to boost your metabolism. Of course, you'll also get other benefits, including increased strength and bone density and improved balance. This beats the side effects of diet pills!
- Add aerobic exercise to burn calories and improve cardiovascular fitness. If you don't enjoy aerobic activity—and it can be painful and unpleasant if you're overweight—give it another try after a month or two of strength training. Don't give up! It's critically important to your health. You'll probably find aerobics easier and more enjoyable when you're stronger.

Q: Can I do this program if I'm pregnant?

A: Guidelines from the American College of Obstetricians and Gynecologists (ACOG) encourage expectant mothers to participate in mild-to-moderate physical exercise. I hope you'll be inspired to become—or remain—active while you're pregnant. However, the ACOG guidelines don't cover strength training. Your joints loosen during pregnancy to help your body prepare for birth—so I don't recommend that you begin this program when you're expecting. If you were strength training prior to conception, ask your doctor if it's safe to continue.

Q: How soon after childbirth can I begin this program?

A: That depends on how quickly your body recovers. Most women feel ready about a month after they give birth—around the time of their postpartum checkup. If you had a cesarean, it's especially important to discuss exercise with your doctor, to make sure your abdominal muscles have healed.

Start at the beginning level (see page 148), even if you've strength-trained before. Increase the weights slowly. Go up every second or third week, paying particular attention to how you feel.

Q: What about kids? Is strength training okay for them? My twelve-year-old daughter is interested, and so is my nine-year-old son.

A: Youngsters can benefit from appropriate strengthening exercise. What's appropriate depends on their age. The American Academy of Pediatrics does not recommend that children age ten and under use free weights or exercise machines. Kids are more prone to injury than adults: They're more likely to drop or trip over weights; and they tend to get impatient and do the moves too quickly. But your son can do strengthening exercises that use body weight: sit-ups, push-ups, pull-ups, stationary jumps, and hill runs.

If there's a suitable program in your area, your daughter might be able to use weights. New evidence suggests that children older than ten can safely strength-train with equipment and will gain important benefits: increased muscle strength and muscle mass, plus improved general fitness. The National Strength and Conditioning Association recently published these safety guidelines for older children who do strength training:

♦ A child should not strength-train without qualified supervision—there should be one instructor for every five to ten children.

- ◆ The instructor should be certified and have experience with children.
- ◆ The child should be physically and emotionally ready, with realistic expectations and strong motivation.
- ◆ Equipment should be in good repair and the proper size for the child.
- ◆ Progress should be very gradual.

Q: I walk nearly an hour a day. Isn't this enough for my bones?

A: I wish more people did what you're doing! Walking is an excellent exercise. Like other aerobic activities, it increases longevity and decreases your risk of chronic diseases. Walking also helps your bones—but it's not enough. In one of my earlier studies, postmenopausal women in a walking program maintained bone density in their spines, but walking didn't benefit their hipbones. Strength training helps both the spine and the hip.

Q: I sit at a desk all day and tend to hunch forward. Will strength training help me?

A: Women who sit at work often have poor posture and back problems—as do those whose jobs keep them on their feet but not moving. Exercises that strengthen the shoulders and upper back will help. (See pages 204 and 205.) Also, if you have a sedentary job, try to be active at other times so you'll stay fit—one simple way is to take brisk walks during lunch breaks. Another is to use the stairs whenever possible.

Q: Will strength training affect how well I do other sports?

A: Yes—and it will reduce the risk of injury too. That's why competitive athletes add strengthening exercises to their regimens. If you're active in a particular sport, be aware that some of your muscles may be very well conditioned while others are not. For instance, a runner may have well-developed legs but untoned arms; a tennis player's racket arm may be muscular, while the other arm is not. So a program that improves overall fitness will be helpful for you.

ADAPTING TO
A MEDICAL CONDITION

Take the PAR-Q (pages 108–109) to find out if you need medical clearance before starting this program. These exercises were developed for elderly men and women, and they're safe for nearly everyone—even individuals with chronic but *stable* medical conditions. Nevertheless, you need to be particularly careful if you have a specific health concern. See page 149 for general guidance, and look at the specific answers below.

Q: **Can I follow this program if I have a bad back?**

A: Talk with your physician. Most people with back problems can do this program—and benefit from it. Start at the beginning level and work up slowly. Concentrate on maintaining good posture as you work out. Be especially careful when you're transporting the weights.

Q: **Will the program relieve my fibromyalgia?**

A: I haven't seen any research on this, but I often hear from women with fibromyalgia who tell me that strength training has helped. Talk to your doctor to make sure it's safe. Proceed conservatively, and listen to your body.

Q: **I have osteoporosis. Is strength training safe for me?**

A: This program was developed for people with this condition, so it's not only safe but beneficial. It is very important to check with your doctor first, though, because you may have special needs. Start the basic program with one-pound weights, and progress slowly, increasing the weight every two or three weeks. Your bones will get stronger as your muscles do, but they need more time. If you want to add exercises for the back and abdomen, talk to your physician; he or she may want to suggest other exercises that are more appropriate.

Q: I've just had a mastectomy. When can I start strength training?

A: Mastectomy, with or without reconstructive surgery, is a major opera-
tion. Some muscle and some lymph nodes may have been removed. Wait six
months before talking to your doctor about starting this program.

If you've ever had a mastectomy, begin this program conservatively.
Your lymphatic system may have been affected by the surgery, and strength
training could cause edema—fluid retention. Start the exercises without
weights, and add weight gradually. Instead of working out at Level 4 intensity, begin with Level 3 (see page 151). Decrease the weights if you notice any
tingling, swelling, or other changes in your chest, shoulder, or arm on the affected side. Once you see that your body is responding positively to the exercises, you can move up to Level 4 and progress normally.

Q: I have arthritis—how will that affect my strength training?

A: My colleague, Ronenn Roubenoff, M.D., has studied the effects of a
high-intensity strength-training program in patients with rheumatoid
arthritis: After twelve weeks they were stronger and their pain was reduced. Some guidelines if you suffer from rheumatoid arthritis or osteoarthritis:

- Don't exercise a joint that is hot and painful. Wait a few
  days, and try again.
- When you do the exercises, work below the pain
  threshold. Progress slowly.
- If you have difficulty holding the hand weights, use wrist
  weights instead—they're available from sporting goods
  stores.

Q: Is it safe to do these exercises if I've had joint-replacement surgery?

A: If you've had a knee or hip replaced, wait until your doctor or physical therapist gives you the go-ahead. Most people are ready to start strength
training six months after surgery, though they may need to work with their
physical therapist to adapt the moves to their needs.

Q: Can I follow this program if I have cardiovascular problems?

A: My colleagues have monitored cardiac patients during strength-training workouts and find that these exercises are safe and beneficial. If you're under a doctor's care for a cardiac problem or high blood pressure, check before you start this program. A reminder: It's especially important to breathe properly when you do the exercises, since holding your breath increases blood pressure.

Q: I have diabetes—will this affect strength training?

A: Several studies have shown that strength training has a special benefit for people with diabetes: It makes the muscles more sensitive to insulin, which can reduce the need for added insulin and help control blood sugar. If you have diabetes, discuss strength training with your doctor before you begin. As with any new exercise, you'll need to monitor your glucose levels closely. An additional caution: Remember to breathe properly when you lift, to avoid increasing vascular pressure.

GETTING READY TO START

Q: I'm eager to begin strength training. But my doctor is discouraging me. He thinks weight lifting is risky for a woman of my age. I'm seventy-eight and in excellent health. What should I do?

A: Please show this book to your doctor, and point out the box on pages 253–254, which lists medical journal articles about the benefits of strength training. Also show him the box on page 149, which suggests ways to adapt this program for women with health concerns. Most doctors become very enthusiastic about strength training once they learn more about it. Indeed, we often hear from physicians—men as well as women—who are following this program themselves!

Do You Have a Hernia? Hemorrhoids? Glaucoma?

If you have these or any other conditions that could be exacerbated by an increase in blood pressure, get clearance from your doctor before you start this program. Proceed cautiously: Start at the beginning level and advance slowly. During your workouts, take care to avoid holding your breath when you lift a heavy weight, since this creates pressure inside your body.

Q: I'm trying to decide if I should do the program with free weights or on machines. Which is better?

A: Both are very beneficial, and I use both myself. The way *you* prefer is best—because that's what you're most likely to stick with. So I suggest you try both and see what you think. You can always switch if you change your mind or if you want some variety.

Q: Do I really need to buy two dumbbells at each weight?

A: You could do the exercises with a single dumbbell and a single leg weight, but each session would take twice as long. The extra time could make the difference between dropping out and sticking with the program. I urge you to get the full set of equipment and find another way to economize—see Chapter 6 for some money-saving suggestions.

Q: Why can't I make weights from milk containers? I've seen directions in a magazine.

A: There are two concerns about do-it-yourself weights. The first is safety. A gallon container isn't designed for weight lifting. The load may not

FOR YOUR DOCTOR

The strength-training program in this book is based on research by our laboratory at the Jean Mayer USDA Human Nutrition Research Center on Aging at Tufts University. The relevant findings were published in these articles:

- Miriam E. Nelson et al., "Effects of High-Intensity Strength Training on Multiple Risk Factors for Osteoporotic Fractures: A Randomized Controlled Trial," *Journal of the American Medical Association* 1994; volume 272, pages 1909–14.
- Maria A. Fiatarone et al., "Exercise Training and Nutritional Supplementation for Physical Frailty in Very Elderly People," *New England Journal of Medicine* 1994; volume 330, pages 1769–75.
- Walter R. Frontera et al., "Strength Conditioning in Older Men: Skeletal Muscle Hypertrophy and Improved Function," *Journal of Applied Physiology* 1988; volume 64, pages 1038–44.

Since this early work was published, many studies from other research centers have documented the benefits of strength training for health. Several comprehensive reviews were published in the January 1999 issue of *Medicine and Science in Sports and Exercise* (volume 31, number 1), including:

- Jennifer Layne and Miriam E. Nelson, "The Effects of Progressive Resistance Training on Bone Density: A Review," pages 25–30.
- William J. Evans, "Exercise Training Guidelines for the Elderly," pages 12–17.

(continued)

♦ David Carpenter and Brian Nelson, "Low Back Strengthening for the Prevention and Treatment of Low Back Pain," pages 18–24.
♦ Neil McCartney, "Acute Responses to Resistance Training and Safety," pages 31–37.
♦ Matthew Feigenbaum and Michael Pollock, "Prescription of Resistance Training for Health and Disease," pages 38–45.

An excellent general review about exercise for older adults is:

♦ Robert Mazzeo et al., "Exercise and Physical Activity for Older Adults," *Medicine and Science in Sports and Exercise* 1998; volume 30, number 6, pages 992–1008.

be balanced, and the container could break if used this way. The second problem is that it's harder to calibrate homemade weights, which means you'll find it more difficult to progress in the gradual way that assures progress without pain or injury.

Q: I'd like to buy a used strength-training machine—any advice?

A: Try before you buy. Make sure the machine is in good repair; check that it fits you. Find out what the machine would cost new to make sure you're getting a good price. See pages 102–103 in Chapter 6.

Q: Can I use a combination of machines and free weights?

A: Yes. Many people add variety to their programs this way. But you'll probably find that even with similar exercises, you'll be lifting different amounts of weight with the home program and the gym program because the equipment isn't the same.

FOLLOWING THE PROGRAM

Q: Can I do one set of all the exercises and then repeat it, or do I have to do two sets of each exercise before moving to the next?

A: I advise doing both sets before you go on to the next exercise. When women do one set, they sometimes never get around to completing the second. The phone rings, a child asks a question—and they don't finish the program.

Q: I'm extremely busy during the week. Can't I do the two sessions on Saturday and Sunday?

A: I don't recommend this. To gain the maximum benefit, you need a day between workouts so your muscles have time to repair themselves. If you do one session over the weekend, you can break the second session into two parts—arms and legs—and slip them in during the week. If there's no other choice, do one session early Saturday and the other late Sunday to give your body the longest possible rest.

Q: How long should I wait after eating before doing the exercises?

A: It's best to wait until you no longer feel full from a meal. Usually that means an hour or more. On the other hand, it's hard to do any kind of exercise on an empty stomach—if you're hungry, all you'll be thinking about is eating.

Q: Is it possible to strength-train too much?

A: Yes. You can push yourself too hard. One sign is that your muscles feel heavy and fatigued during the day. They shouldn't. Never strength-train the same muscle more than three times a week, because you'll be much more prone to injury. Your muscles need time to rest and repair—this is when they actually get stronger.

How Many Sets and Reps are Enough?

Readers often ask me about research done at the University of Florida and elsewhere, which compared the results of strength training with one, two, or three sets. Investigators found that one set was just as effective as two or three in increasing muscle strength. In part because of this research, the American College of Sports Medicine (ACSM) issued the following position statement in 1998: "One set of eight to ten exercises that conditions the major muscle groups two to three days per week is recommended. Multiple-set regimens may provide greater benefits if time allows." Both the research and the ACSM recommendations have been reported in many popular publications.

We're all pressed for time, so it's tempting to cut back on workouts. But before you drop the second set, you need to know some important limitations of the findings. The University of Florida study, like others that have obtained similar results, put volunteers on regimens that were different from the *Strong Women* program in two important respects:

First, each workout involved ten or more different exercises, so each major muscle group was worked by at least two exercises.

Second, these programs used strength-training machines, not free weights (dumbbells and ankle weights). Machines hold your body in the correct position, which usually allows you to lift heavier weights.

What does this mean for you?

If you're following the gym version of the *Strong Women Stay Young* program, which calls for ten exercises, the research suggests that you complete two sets to get the most out of your workout. This is consistent with the ACSM recommendation, which says that multiple sets may provide more benefit.

If you are following the at-home exercise plan and have added supplemental moves so your workout includes more than twelve exercises, you could cut back to one set of eight exercises if time is a problem. However, if you're doing just eight exercises, I still recommend that you complete two sets of eight repetitions to get the full benefit for your muscles and bones.

Q: I want to do aerobics and strength training—how do I combine them?

A: The usual recommendation for aerobics is to work out for thirty minutes three to six days a week. Be sure to take one day off each week to assure that your body has time to rest and repair. You can add a complete strength-training program to your workout two or three of those days, or you can add a few strengthening exercises every day, so long as you don't work the same muscle two days in a row. I suggest you do the aerobic exercise first, to warm your muscles for strength training.

Q: I can easily lift eight pounds in the overhead press with my right arm but can barely manage it with my left arm. Should I use a heavier weight for my right arm, or should I continue and wait for the left arm to catch up?

A: Advance more slowly—every other week—with your stronger arm. But since it's better for both sides of your body to be equal in strength, try to progress every week with your weaker arm to help it catch up.

Q: Sometimes my muscle trembles during a workout. Should I be concerned about that?

A: No—it simply means your muscle is working at high intensity. You're most likely to see muscle trembling when you've recently increased the amount of weight you're lifting; it usually happens after you've done several

DO YOU GET ENOUGH PROTEIN?

Most Americans get plenty of protein in their diets without any special effort. If you're following the guidelines in the Food Guide Pyramid (page 34) you don't need to increase your protein because you're strength training. Nor is it desirable for you to take protein supplements. There is no evidence that adding protein supplements to an adequate diet will enhance the benefits of strength training. But certain individuals should pay extra attention to make sure they meet their protein needs:

- **Vegetarians who don't eat eggs or dairy foods (vegans)**
  Most Americans get their protein from meat, eggs, dairy products, beans, and grains. Vegans—who don't eat any animal products—*can* get sufficient protein from grains and beans, but they must select carefully. (For further information, see the list of recommended nutrition books on page 41.)

- **People with eating disorders**
  Individuals who starve themselves, or those who are caught in a cycle of bingeing and purging, often don't consume enough protein (or they consume but don't digest it). Similarly, an extremely restricted diet—either very low in calories or very limited in food choices, such as an all-grapefruit diet—may not supply adequate protein.

- **The elderly**
  About a quarter of people over age fifty-five do not get enough protein. Some have physical or emotional problems that affect their eating habits; others don't choose foods well or can't afford a proper diet.

repetitions. Since trembling occurs when the weight is a challenge, just be sure that you haven't moved ahead too quickly: You should be lifting a weight that you can lift eight times *in good form.*

Q: I hear weird noises—grinding, popping—in my knee when I do the knee extension. What does this mean?

A: Grinding noises are made when rough cartilage on the end of one bone rubs against cartilage on the end of another bone in your joint. People with osteoarthritis or previous knee injuries are most likely to hear or feel grinding. As long as the exercise is not painful, it's safe to proceed.

A popping sound indicates that a ligament or tendon—connective tissue attached to bone—has realigned itself over the joint. It's most likely to happen during the first repetition of a lift. If it doesn't hurt, don't worry about it.

TROUBLESHOOTING

Q: I really want to follow this program, but I'm very busy, and sometimes two weeks go by between workouts. Any suggestions?

A: This is a common problem. The best solution is to make training sessions part of your weekly routine. One way to fix a routine is to have a regular appointment to work out with a friend. Another is to do the exercises while you watch a television program that you never miss. See Chapter 10 for more suggestions.

Q: A five-pound dumbbell isn't enough of a challenge, but I can't do all the lifts when I jump to the next dumbbell, which is eight pounds. What should I do?

A: Make the transition gradually. Do the first set with five pounds and then move up to eight pounds for the second set. If this still doesn't work, purchase a six- or seven-pound dumbbell to make the change easier.

"I Lose Track When I Count"

This isn't a serious problem—your body won't know the difference if occasionally you do seven repetitions, or nine, instead of the prescribed eight. A few tricks to help:

- ♦ Count out loud: This helps you keep track and guarantees that you breathe properly.
- ♦ Use your fingers: Pick a method and use it consistently. Mine is to keep track with four fingers on one hand, counting off twice for each set.
- ♦ Take turns: If you're in a group, one person can keep track while everyone talks.

Q: I'm doing the program with a friend who's my age. She's moving ahead much more quickly, and I'm becoming discouraged.

A: Keep going! Try to focus on the progress you're making. Where you start and how fast you improve depend on your initial level of fitness, your health, and other individual factors. I bet you and your friend end up at about the same point, even if it takes you a little longer to get there.

Q: I've been doing the program for a few months, and my wrists are really sore. Am I doing something wrong? How can I resolve this, so I can continue strength training?

A: The problem could be your form; or it could be that your wrists are weak. If so, one or more of these suggestions should help:

WRIST CURLS

Strengthen your wrists with this simple exercise. Stronger wrists are useful for more than lifting dumbbells—especially if your job involves typing, data entry, or other activities that can cause repetitive motion injuries.

Start with one- or two-pound dumbbells. Sit in a chair, with your feet flat on the floor, shoulder-width apart. Hold one weight in each hand. Lean slightly forward and rest your forearms on your thighs. Your wrists should be slightly beyond your knees with palms facing up.

- **1-2-3-Lower:** Bend your wrists to slowly lower the back of your hands toward your shins.
- **Pause** for a breath.
- **1-2-3-Raise:** Slowly bring your palms back up, until your wrists are straight again.
- **Pause** for a breath and repeat. Do one set of eight reps.

For the second set of eight reps, turn your hands over: Keep your forearms on your thighs but with your palms facing down. As you do the second set, your wrists will bend forward, not back.

Note: Your forearms never lose contact with your thighs during the lifts. Only your wrists move, not your forearm or upper arm.

- Make sure that your wrists stay straight and in line with your forearm when you're doing the upper-body exercises, particularly the biceps curl and overhead press.
- Wear wrist braces for a little additional support.
- To strengthen your wrists, do wrist curls (see box above).

If—despite these measures—the pain continues, please see your doctor promptly. There could be a physical problem that needs to be addressed.

Q: I'm forty-eight years old and have been strength-training for two months now. I have pain in my hip joints when doing the side hip raises. It doesn't seem to make any difference how much or how little weight I use—the pain is the same. Is there any way to modify this movement?

A: From time to time, I hear from a reader who is experiencing pain from the exercises. It's clear she's not talking about the fleeting discomfort of muscle fatigue—"good" pain that's normal during a high-intensity strengthening workout. Nor is it the mild soreness that beginners may feel after the first few workouts. My answer is the same, whether the problem is in the hip or elsewhere in the body: Discontinue the exercises that give you pain, and see your primary care physician to have the problem checked. You should not experience acute pain or discomfort with exercise. If you do, that could indicate a medical problem. Only after you rule out such a problem should you look for alternative exercises.

Q: I've been following the program for ten months and seem to have reached my limit. What do I do now for maintenance?

A: Just keep strength-training twice a week. You needn't attempt to increase the weights, but I suggest you swap exercises periodically. You'll work more muscles, and your program will remain fresh.

AFTERWORD

Now that you've finished the book, I hope you're well on your way to becoming stronger. Perhaps you've begun the exercises, or maybe you're still thinking about it.

I have great confidence that you'll succeed, because I've seen it happen so often. The women in my *JAMA* study were sedentary when they started. After strength training, all of them became more active—and almost all of them have remained so even now that the study is over. They tell us they're stronger than they have ever been in their lives. At an age when many of their peers are slowing down, these women have renewed energy and the excitement of new opportunities.

I wish you that same strength, vitality, and empowerment.

INDEX

ABOUT MIRIAM NELSON AND
SARAH WERNICK

Authors of *Strong Women Stay Young*
and *Strong Women Stay Slim*

Miriam Nelson, Ph.D., is Director of the Center for Physical Fitness at the School of Nutrition Science and Policy at Tufts University. She is a Fellow of the American College of Sports Medicine and holds their certification as a health/fitness director. She is lead author or coauthor on original research papers that have been published in distinguished peer-reviewed journals, including *Journal of the American Medical Association* and *New England Journal of Medicine*. In 1994 she was named a Brookdale National Fellow. This prestigious award is given annually to only five or six young scholars in the field of aging. She was a 1997–98 Bunting Fellow at the Mary Ingraham Bunting Institute at Radcliffe College. She lives in Concord, Massachusetts, with her husband and three children.

Sarah Wernick, Ph.D., is an award-winning freelance writer based in Brookline, Massachusetts, who specializes in health and family issues. She is married and has two children.

The *Strong Women Stay Young* Web site is http://www.strongwomen.com

The *Strong Women Stay Young* video is available from Women First Health-Care. The video, based on the first edition of this book, features Miriam Nelson, Ph.D., with fitness trainer Bonnie Falbo, P.A. For more information, call toll free 1-888-7-WOMEN-1.